10,000 STEPS A DAY IN L.A.

52 WALKING ADVENTURES

by Paul Haddad

SANTA
MONICA
PRESS

Published by:
Santa Monica Press LLC
P.O. Box 850
Solana Beach, CA 92075
1-800-784-9553
www.santamonicapress.com
books@santamonicapress.com

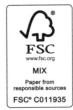

Printed in the United States

Santa Monica Press books are available at special quantity discounts when purchased in bulk by corporations, organizations, or groups. Please call our Special Sales department at 1-800-784-9553.

This book is intended to provide general information. The publisher, author, distributor, and copyright owner are not engaged in rendering professional advice or services. The publisher, author, distributor, and copyright owner are not liable or responsible to any person or group with respect to any loss, illness, or injury caused or alleged to be caused by the information found in this book.

ISBN-13 978-1-59580-084-8

Library of Congress Cataloging-in-Publication Data

Haddad, Paul.
10,000 steps a day in L.A. : 52 walking adventures / by Paul Haddad.
    pages cm
  Summary: "The first book to integrate the '10,000 steps' fitness phenomenon into the Los Angeles terrain, 10,000 Steps a Day in L.A. : 52 Walking Adventures takes readers through the beaches, mountains, parks, rivers, and reservoirs of L.A. while immersing them in the city's lore, history, landmarks, and sometimes quirky locales"--Provided by publisher.
  ISBN 978-1-59580-084-8
  1. Los Angeles (Calif.)--Tours. 2. Walking--California--Los Angeles--Guidebooks. 3. Physical fitness--California--Los Angeles. I. Title. II. Title: Ten thousand steps a day in Los Angeles. III. Title: Ten thousand steps a day in L.A. IV. Title: 10,000 steps a day in Los Angeles.
  F869.L83H23 2015
  979.4'94--dc23
                        2015010819

Cover and interior design and production by Future Studio
Maps by Bryan Duddles
Photos by Paul Haddad

CONTENTS

HOLLYWOOD AND MID-CITY

WEST SAN GABRIEL VALLEY

SAN FERNANDO VALLEY

WESTSIDE

SOUTH BAY

GREETINGS, WALKER!

Since you made the decision to pick up this book, you are obviously a walking apostle. You're in good company. Some of humanity's greatest minds—from Ludwig van Beethoven to President Truman to Steve Jobs—enjoyed daily constitutionals. And since you live in the twenty-first century, chances are you're the owner of a pedometer, a Fitbit, or some other digital doohickey that measures your steps on a daily basis. (And if you don't own one, no worries—you can still do these walks without one.)

For many of us, 10,000 steps a day has become our mantra. The concept first took hold in Japan in the 1960s. Dr. Yoshiro Hatano determined that a person who takes 10,000 steps a day would burn twenty percent of their caloric intake. To this day, a pedometer in Japan is called a *manpo-kei* (literally, "10,000 steps meter").

Flash-forward to the present. The benefits of 10,000 daily steps are hailed by a number of health institutions: the World Health Organization (WHO), the U.S. Center for Disease Control, the American Heart Foundation, and the U.S. Department of Health and Human Services. Companies like Kaiser Permanente and the Mayo Clinic have joined health experts Dr. Oz and Bob Greene (Oprah's trainer) and a growing list of celebrities in publicly endorsing the 10,000-steps program. On a local level, friends of my wife and mine are known to display their daily steps to one another with the same gushing pride once reserved for pictures of their kids. I've personally become so obsessed that I'll sometimes pace my living room before bed just to rack up the steps needed to get to that magical five-digit number. Hey, at least I don't have a tread-mill desk. Yet.

Attaining 10,000 daily steps is a reminder that staying active as an adult takes work, especially in a car-centric city like Los Angeles. I'm a native myself, having come of age in the canyons below Mulholland Drive. Rambling the hills behind our house until dusk, I never worried about fitness milestones. Apparently, grown-ups didn't much either. My father's favorite pastime was taking the family out for Sunday drives. This was around the same time that the new wave band Missing Persons was telling us "nobody walks in L.A." You don't hear the phrase "Sunday drive" much anymore, and the cliché about no one walking here is as passé as jokes about our smog. Welcome to twenty-first-century Los Angeles, where "road diet" and "walkability index" are the new buzzwords.

What accounts for our budding love affair with our feet? Many things—strong communities built around younger families, millennials moving into urban digs, city planners pushing transit-oriented projects, and a renewed awareness of nature and the environment. All of these are byproducts of healthy living. Long walks make us feel good; without them, our day feels incomplete.

Still, some days 10,000 steps prove elusive. Your boss keeps you late at the office. The kids have karate practice. The cable guy gave you a four-hour window and he's *still* running late. But there's always the weekend. For many of us, Sunday drives have been replaced by weekend jaunts or hikes, when we can carve out more time to seek out our surroundings than during the work week. It's why this book is broken up into fifty-two walks—one for each weekend of the year. Which leads to another aspect of walking, perhaps the most important of all, because without it, we wouldn't want to do it in the first place:

Walking should be *fun*.

I may be biased, but I believe there is no greater walkable metropolis than Los Angeles. My observation has been

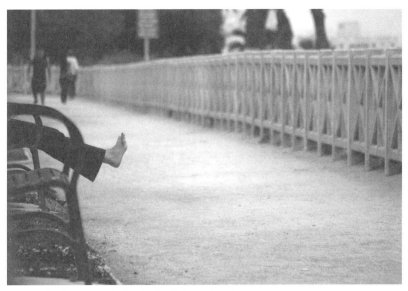

Letting the dogs out at Palisades Park, Santa Monica.

shaped by a lifetime of exploring L.A. and traveling to forty-eight other states and thirty countries. Like Manhattan, we have our own cultural enclaves marked by historic architecture and exotic cuisine. But we are also blessed with a temperate climate and a famously diverse topography that includes a swath of mountains right through the center of the city. We also have Hollywood. Whether it's moseying through an old Western movie set, circling TV's most famous fishing hole, or dropping by not one but *both* churches where future president Ronald Reagan married his two wives, this book trains our pedometers on L.A.'s unique and endlessly fascinating stature as the entertainment capital of the world.

That's not to say you should expect to plant your heels in Tom Cruise's footprints at the Chinese Theatre. These walks favor the obscure over the obvious. They retrace the routes of a proposed freeway and an old bicycle tollway, revisit the haunts of abandoned neighborhoods and amusement parks, and pay tribute to the legions of dreamers lured by the

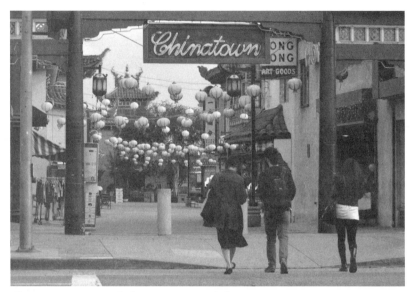

The Western Gateway of Chinatown's Central Plaza.

promise of the Golden State but whose dreams went unrealized. Of course, many dreamers made good on their grandiose visions—Hubert Eaton, Abbot Kinney, Griffith J. Griffith, and Ray "Crash" Corrigan, to name a few—and they're celebrated in these pages, too. And though some tourist traps are unavoidable, they're presented in a context that helps explain what made them cultural touchstones in the first place.

Of course, modern Los Angeles owes its very existence to imported water, a complex saga that inspired *Chinatown* and continues to define who we are. More than one-third of the journeys in this book take you to our city's lakes, arroyos, reservoirs, hidden creeks, or flood control basins. Besides separating history from revisionist history, these waterly walks reveal unexpected oases that shimmer in the sunlight and connect us to the land.

Ultimately, *all* of these walks are about connectivity. At 472 square miles, Los Angeles can be an overwhelming place. But it doesn't have to be. Like a giant piñata, L.A. works best when you crack open its papier-mâché exterior and revel in its panoply of flavors. With that in mind, these fifty-two routes extend to all four corners of the city—from Pasadena to Pacific Palisades, and Chatsworth to Baldwin Hills—and cover fourteen more municipalities either within or just beyond its borders.

Once you get a few dozen treks under your feet, an interesting thing starts to happen. Linkages form from one community to the next. And although they retain singular identities, taken together, they tell the narrative of Los Angeles in all its messy, chewy goodness.

Before you venture out and tackle the city step by step, here are a few ground rules to keep in mind:

Not all 10,000 steps are created equal. I'm a shade over the average height of an American male (about five feet ten inches). Taller people have longer strides, shorter people have shorter ones. My stride equals one mile for every 2,000 steps. Your steps may have to be moderately calibrated—check your pedometer's instructions. One figure you can depend on: each walk is approximately five miles.

The best things in life are free . . . except when they're not. These itineraries purposely avoid routes where you have to pay for access (sorry, Descanso Gardens). However, there are occasional museums you may want to visit along the way. I also tried to choose starting points that allow for free street parking, though that's not always possible in denser neighborhoods.

Go Metro. Forty-six of the fifty-two tours are within walking distance of Metro bus stops. Seventeen are within a few blocks of a Metro rail line or busway. If you prefer not to drive to each walk's starting point, check out your public transit options at www.metro.net.

Keep your eyes wide open. I'm always amazed at the new things I pick up whenever I repeat a walk. For example, FDR's Works Progress Administration shaped much of the

Southland's landscape in the '30s and '40s. Its art and engineering projects pop up like Easter eggs where you least expect them. My role here is tour guide, but I'm hardly the last word. To paraphrase a famous author, feel free to throw off the bowlines on occasion and chart your own path. Consider the maps that accompany each walk your safe harbor to get you back on track.

Bring a (furry) friend. We have a hyperactive family member who takes tens of thousands of steps a day. Of course, it helps to have four legs. His name is Porter, and he was my walking buddy for many of these itineraries. Yep, that's him in the pictures. If you're a dog lover, you know how they can make the simplest walk more fun (squirrels may disagree). Still, some of these routes are not geared for dogs, often because they aren't allowed on certain premises. Check the "Fido Friendly?" line at the beginning of each chapter. Note that you will have to leash your dog if you go inside some buildings.

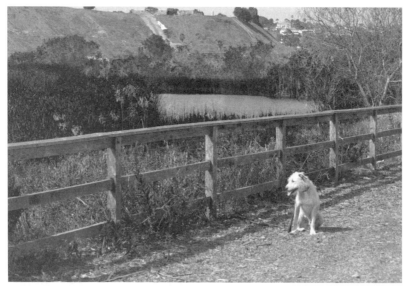

My trusty walking companion, Porter, takes a breather during a "Fido Friendly" walk at Ballona Wetlands.

A pair of comfortable shoes will do. Remember, these are walks—sturdy hiking shoes are not necessary. But to keep things interesting, we do sometimes tread on dirt paths. Since you're already logging 10,000 steps, I try to steer clear of long, extended hills. You can find terrain information at the beginning of each chapter.

Don't forget to exercise your mouth, too. Every workout needs a reward. If you're the picnicking type, or if you brought your dog, feel free to pack a meal. I've included optimal "Picnic Ops" for every walk. Then again, your nose will quickly alert you to several culinary landmarks that you'll pass. Who can resist a pastrami sandwich at Langer's, or the taco variety plate from Guisados? (My mouth is watering just writing those words.) With the exception of two treks into the Hollywood Hills, each itinerary also includes suggestions where chowhounds can get a taste of authentic L.A. fare.

One reason 10,000 daily steps is so appealing is that it involves a fixed target, akin to conquering a mountain or running a 10K. By adding a treasure-hunt element, my goal is to give you, the intrepid urban adventurer, an even deeper appreciation for our hometown while simultaneously making 10,000 steps go by that much faster. So strap on your sneaks, calibrate your *manpo-kei*, and get out there and enjoy the City of Angels! I'll see you in another half-million or so steps.

PAUL HADDAD
Los Angeles, CA

Overleaf: The downtown L.A. skyline from Vista Hermosa Park.

CENTRAL L.A. AND THE EASTSIDE

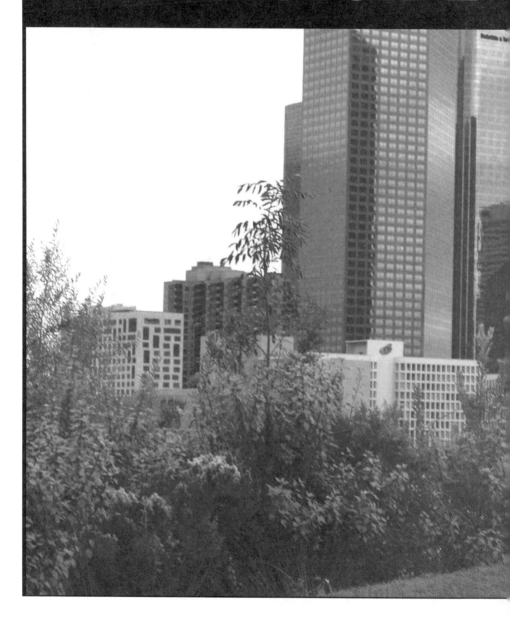

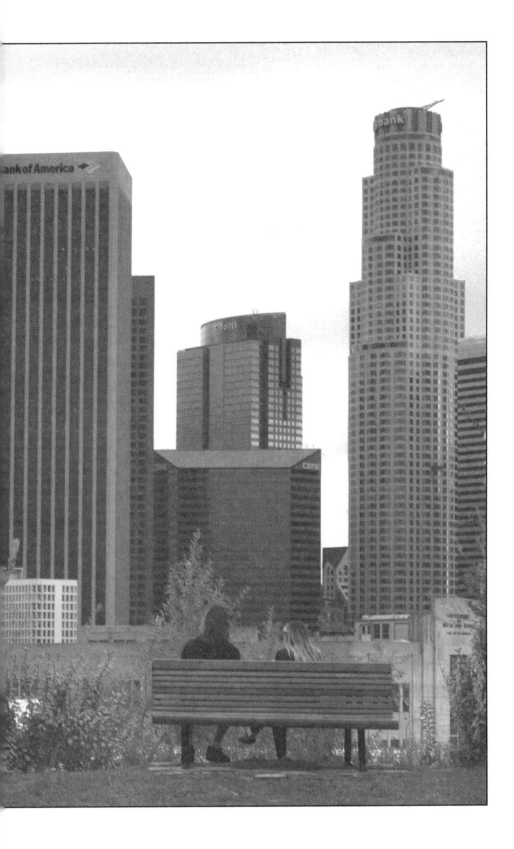

1

DOWNTOWN LOS ANGELES

THIS WAY TO PEDWAYS!

This walk through central L.A. crosses time and space, refracting over 100 years of change that inspire, fascinate, and sometimes just baffle—as in the case of its bridges to insignificance.

- **TERRAIN:** Flat with stairs and minimal inclines
- **SURFACE:** Paved
- **FIDO FRIENDLY?:** No (multiple interior premises)
- **PARKING:** Several lots near Civic Center/Grand Park Metro Station, at 101 Hill Street, Los Angeles

Downtown Los Angeles is an urban receptacle of awful ideas. Blame post-WWII suburbanization for most of them. The city's core was reimagined as an autotopia, with pedestrians redirected off streets to bridges above the fray. All this poor planning left downtown ill-prepared for the influx of residents moving back in, many of them happily carless.

Fortunately for us walkers, follies make for fun counterparts to the dignified landmarks that have managed to withstand decades of change. **Start at the Metro station on Hill Street,** which slices through Grand Park. **Head through the park toward Spring Street, just a couple blocks east.** The twelve-acre park has been an unexpected hit since it first opened, injecting much-needed vibrancy and green space to L.A.'s soulless Civic Center. Even when there aren't public events, there's a lot to sample here. Sure, Grand Park will never match the cultural magnitude of New York's Central Park,

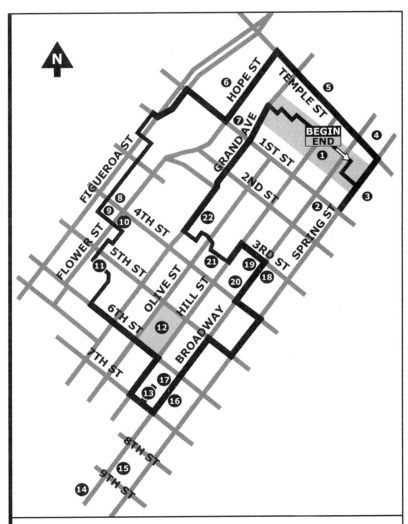

1. GRAND PARK
2. L.A. TIMES BUILDING
3. CITY HALL
4. HALL OF JUSTICE
5. CATHEDRAL OF OUR LADY OF THE ANGELS
6. DEPARTMENT OF WATER AND POWER
7. MUSIC CENTER
8. WORLD TRADE CENTER
9. BONAVENTURE HOTEL
10. YMCA BUILDING
11. CENTRAL LIBRARY
12. PERSHING SQUARE
13. SAINT VINCENT COURT
14. UNITED ARTISTS THEATRE
15. ORPHEUM THEATRE
16. PALACE THEATRE
17. LOS ANGELES THEATRE
18. BRADBURY BUILDING
19. MILLION DOLLAR THEATER
20. GRAND CENTRAL MARKET
21. ANGELS FLIGHT
22. CALIFORNIA PLAZA

but it's the closest thing
we have to a downtown
gathering place, an open
letter to elected officials
that shouts, "Dear L.A.: More like this!"

PICNIC OP
Grand Park, between Grand Avenue and Hill Street.

Arriving at Spring Street, go one block south to 1st Street. Catty-corner from where you're standing is the Los Angeles Times Building, which bears an intentional resemblance to a fortress. A block away, an early Los Angeles Times edifice was blown up by anti-union activists in 1910, killing over twenty people. Possible remnants of the old headquarters were discovered in 2014 during Grand Park's expansion.

Head north up Spring. On your right you'll see City Hall, for decades the tallest high-rise in Los Angeles. A little-known observation deck on the twenty-seventh floor is open to the public on weekdays.

Turn left on Temple Street, passing the Hall of Justice on your right. The 1926 courthouse of white Sierra granite has a distinctive colonnade on its upper levels. Bugsy Siegel, Charles Manson, Sirhan Sirhan, O. J. Simpson—L.A.'s baddest bad boys have paraded through here. Another two blocks brings you to the Cathedral of Our Lady of the Angels. The Catholic church's sun-baked color is an ode to the old California missions. Note the building's avoidance of right angles, which the church believes "contributes to the Cathedral's feeling of mystery."

Turn left at Hope Street and look to the right. No, you're not dreaming. The Department of Water and Power Building starred in the dream sequences in *Inception*. Both it and the Music Center complex on the left betray their 1960s origins in their designs and ambitions. As replacements for the Victorian-era homes that used to dot this hillside, they signified a new, modern direction for downtown.

Cross 1st Street and make a right. After one block, turn left, following the sidewalk down the ramp with

a "Do Not Enter" sign (the exit lane for automobiles leaving Figueroa Street). At 2nd Street, cross over to the west side of Figueroa and continue south. Halfway down the block, you'll come to a pedestrian bridge overhead. **Access the overpass by taking the stairway up** (it's tucked between a column and a driveway). You are about to enter an odd journey. For this is not just any bridge, but a bridge to the Twilight Zone of Misguided Urban Planning.

The elevated pedestrian walkway, or pedway, is one of ten that were built in the 1970s, crisscrossing a nine-block section of downtown at random places. This pedway parallels Figueroa and leads to a circular plaza, where you'll find a pedway map and plaque dedicated to Calvin S. Hamilton, the city's former director of planning. Removing pesky pedestrians from the city's mean streets must have seemed like a good idea back when downtowns across America were in decline. But Hamilton's vision didn't stop there—Phase Two was going to equip the pedways with people-movers like Disneyland used to have. Funding ran out before Hamilton's Mickey Mouse project could be completed, but that doesn't mean we can't retrace his good intentions.

Continue along the pedway over 3rd Street. It leads to a deserted, unassuming courtyard belonging to the World Trade Center—a far cry from what one would expect from such a prodigious organization. **Enter the glass doors,** to the left of a stairway that leads to roof-top tennis courts. Once inside, look up and find an impressive frieze titled "History of Commerce" spanning the otherwise moribund northern lobby.

Find the escalator at the southern exit and take it up to another pedway. This one crosses 4th Street, leading to the northern entrance of the futuristic Bonaventure Hotel— or at least, the future as envisioned in the 1970s. Inside, the hotel's massive atrium is a confusing warren of glass elevators, spiral stairways, and swirling hallways leading to lonely shops that, like a mirage, always seem to elude your grasp.

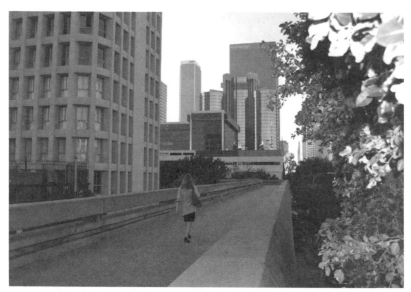

A businesswoman strikes a lonely figure on a downtown pedway.

Perhaps this disorientation is what really led to John Malkovich's climactic demise in this hotel in the 1993 Clint Eastwood movie *In the Line of Fire*.

Take a stairwell or elevator up to the sixth floor, following signs that say "Bridge to YMCA & Arco Garage." Exit the hotel's eastern face and you will find yourself on another pedway, this one the highest of them all. Imagine soaring above Flower Street on a cushion of air in your own puttering people-pod. No, I can't imagine it either.

Crossing over to the YMCA concourse, hang a right and find the elevator for the parking garage on the left side. Hop in the elevator and press the button for the seventh floor, which is accompanied by the anticipatory words "Bonaventure Sky Bridge." When the doors open on the seventh floor, **turn right and cross said "sky bridge" back to the Bonaventure. Instead of entering the hotel again, stay on the pedway as it turns left and soars over 5th Street.** A stairway takes you down to the southwest corner of 5th and Flower. Thanks to the pedways, you've just walked two and a half blocks without touching a sidewalk . . . though it probably took you twice as long!

Cross over to the Central Library on the east side of Flower. The 1926 compound's roof contains a tiled mosaic of a sun in a pyramid, reflecting the "Light of Learning." The library is fronted by the beautifully landscaped Maguire Gardens. **Stroll through the gardens to the library's southern entrance and take the stairs down to Hope Street**, turning right.

Next, turn left on 6th Street. In two blocks, you'll come to Pershing Square. Once populated by trees and trails, the park was "updated" in the 1950s. At the same time car-happy planners were ripping out streetcar lines, they replaced Pershing Square's grass with concrete and added a parking garage down below, cutting the park off from the street. Still, Pershing remains a welcome respite amidst downtown's towers, and plans are underway to restore its accessibility.

Turn right on Hill, then left on 7th Street. Halfway down the block, make a left into Saint Vincent Court, a kitschy pedestrian-only alley that dates back 100 years and is now a California State Landmark. After checking out its faux-Old World charms, **turn left on 7th and then left on Broadway.** At 615 is the Los Angeles Theatre, a French Baroque gem from 1931—the last of the ornate movie palaces built downtown. Its opening night movie? The world premiere of Charlie Chaplin's *City Lights*.

Turn right on 5th Street. On the northwest corner of 5th and Spring

EXTRA STEPS

From 1910 to the early '30s, Broadway was the center of cinematic grandeur, with twelve movie palaces covering a six-block stretch. Most of the remaining theaters can be viewed between 7th and 3rd Streets, including the refurbished United Artists, Orpheum, and Palace. The Los Angeles Conservancy hosts tours and occasional screenings.

is the Last Bookstore, whose second-floor décor is downright Seussian—it must be seen to be believed.

Continue north on Spring. Go left on 4th Street, then right on Broadway. At the end of the block is the Bradbury Building. Though it remains a commercial-tenant building—the oldest in downtown L.A.—visitors are allowed on the ground floor. Its open-cage elevators, glass ceiling, and iron railings are living fossils of the Victorian Age. Paradoxically, the building nicely represented the "future" in the movie *Blade Runner*. (P.S.: Don't miss the Charlie Chaplin figure sitting on a bench in the back. The Tramp lived a block away, in the historic El Dorado Building.)

Cross the street to the Million Dollar Theater. You might recognize Sid Grauman's first movie house from the movie *(500) Days of Summer*. Next to it is Grand Central Market, taking up the ground floor of a terracotta structure built in 1896. Grab some grub at any of its bustling market stalls offering a range of worldly cuisines.

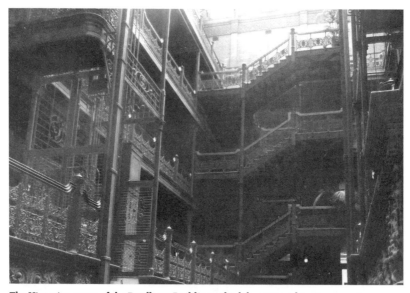

The Victorian court of the Bradbury Building, which has starred in many movies.

Exit Grand Central Market from its western portal and take the crosswalk across Hill to Angels Flight, a true civic treasure. For over 100 years, the funicular railway shuttled passengers up and down Bunker Hill. But mechanical problems have plagued the historic landmark, causing intermittent closures. If you find it shuttered, simply make do as nineteenth-century denizens did—up the flight of 153 steps to the left of the railway!

Once at the top, you'll stumble upon a pond and courtyard between two skyscrapers that make up California Plaza, also home to the Museum of Contemporary Art. **Head west through the courtyard,** which lets out on Grand Avenue. **Turn right on Grand and proceed to Grand Park** (half a block north of 1st Street). **Walk through the park to either the Metro train or the parking lot,** where your glorified people-mover awaits to shuttle you back home.

2

CHINATOWN / OLVERA STREET / LITTLE TOKYO

DOWNTOWN'S CULTURAL TRIANGLE

This route connects three historic points in northern downtown, including the celebrated birthplace of El Pueblo de la Reina de Los Angeles—"L.A." to you and me.

- **TERRAIN:** Flat with stairs
- **SURFACE:** Mostly paved
- **FIDO FRIENDLY?:** Yes
- **PARKING:** Lot in Bamboo Plaza, at 420 Bernard Street, Chinatown

When it comes to Los Angeles's Historic-Cultural Monuments, preservation often takes a back seat to progress. So Victorian homes get uprooted for skyscrapers and plopped in Heritage Square. An iconic hot dog stand that looks like a hot dog gets wheeled from one street to another to make room for condos. When the city wanted to build Union Station where the original Chinatown stood, it simply bulldozed the entire neighborhood and re-built it in a new location. Even Los Angeles itself was founded not at Olvera Street, but at a site near the L.A. River. Only Little Tokyo retains its original boundaries, though Japanese Americans weren't always around to enjoy it. After being interned in camps during World War II, it took decades for many to return. All that aside, the proximity of these ethnic districts to one another makes for a colorful and vibrant walk that exemplifies L.A.'s melting pot.

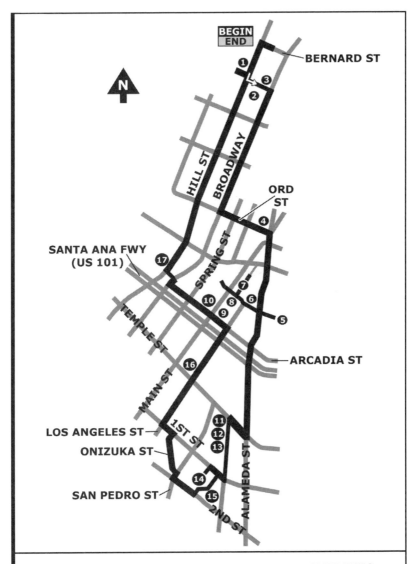

1. WEST PLAZA
2. CENTRAL PLAZA
3. PHOENIX BAKERY
4. PHILIPPE
5. UNION STATION
6. PASEO DE LA PLAZA
7. OLVERA STREET
8. LOS ANGELES PLAZA PARK
9. PICO HOUSE
10. OUR LADY QUEEN OF THE ANGELS CATHOLIC CHURCH
11. GO FOR BROKE MONUMENT
12. GEFFEN CONTEMPORARY AT MOCA
13. JAPANESE AMERICAN NATIONAL MUSEUM
14. KOYASAN BUDDHIST TEMPLE
15. JAPANESE VILLAGE PLAZA
16. LOS ANGELES MALL
17. FORT MOORE PIONEER MEMORIAL

Start on the north side of Bernard Street, between Hill Street and Broadway in Chinatown. In the middle of the block are two small Victorian-era houses. They're owned by the Chinese Heritage and Visitors Center, which possesses a collection of artifacts dug up from the original Chinatown.

Continue west on Bernard, turning left on Hill. On your right you'll see West Plaza, a 1948 courtyard crowned by rows of Chinese lanterns. Note the informational kiosk with historical photos—one of many that can be found along this triangular itinerary. Discover the plaza's hidden alleyways and polychromatic staircases leading up to the back doors of second-story apartments.

Leaving West Plaza, take the crosswalk to the east side of Hill. Walk through the historic West Gate to Central Plaza, one of four gates in the district. Linger at the plaza's kitschy shops and monuments. Momentarily freak out at the sound of small explosions, only to realize it's just kids slamming gunpowder-filled caps onto the ground. The architectural high point here is the five-tiered pagoda that makes up the Hop Louie restaurant, built in 1941. A newer addition to the square is the Bruce Lee statue by the Eastern Gate, clutching nunchucks and looking badass.

Exit the Eastern Gate and turn left up Broadway. In just a few steps, you'll encounter the seventy-five-year-old Phoenix Bakery, with its chubby Chinese boy beckoning for more "sweets for the sweet."

Turn around and head back down Broadway, turning left on Ord Street. Pause at Ord and Spring Street and conjure up the ending of the 1974 noir thriller *Chinatown*. The final bloody scene where Nicholson is told, "Forget it, Jake, it's Chinatown" took place near this intersection. (As for the movie's fictionalized version of L.A.'s water history, well, never let the truth get in the way of a good story.)

Proceed one more block to Ord and Alameda Street. There are several awesome culinary choices along this route, but if you want a true original, Philippe has been cranking out French-dipped sandwiches since 1908. Step inside its sawdust-covered floor and order at the counter. Though they serve 300 pounds of pigs' feet a week, I'll stick with my usual—a double-dip turkey sandwich with Swiss cheese!

Just south of Philippe, cross Alameda at Main Street. Continue south on the east sidewalk—past the double-domed Mission Revival building that used to be L.A.'s main post office—and soak in the splendor of Union Station, the last great train terminal built in the United States. Enter the cathedral-like waiting room and go gaga over the ornate details of its expansive interior. Wander inside and plop into an oversized leather chair. Yes, those are pigeons flying near the ceiling. To really do this 1939 landmark justice, schedule a Los Angeles Conservancy tour, which takes you into rooms now closed to the public, including the original ticket lobby.

Departing the station, proceed across Alameda to the northwest corner of Alameda and Los Angeles Street. This is the entrance to Paseo De La Plaza, the all-encompassing term for the array of old buildings, alleyways, museums, and memorials that mark L.A.'s Hispanic heritage. **Start with Olvera Street, to your immediate right.** As you survey its souvenir stands, be sure to glance down, too, where the zigzag designs of Olvera's brick surface retrace the original path of the Zanja Madre (the "Mother Ditch" we now know as the Los Angeles River). Duck into Avila Adobe; at almost 200 years old, it's the oldest surviving residence in Los Angeles and contains many relics from the city's early years.

At the end of Olvera Street, turn around and head out the way you came. South of the street is Los Angeles Plaza Park, marked by a gazebo and statues of King Carlos III of Spain, Father Junipero Serra, and other luminaries. The plaza dates back to 1820, symbolizing the

PICNIC OP

Los Angeles Plaza Park, 125 Paseo De La Plaza.

city's (erroneous) birthplace. Just south of the park are several historic buildings, including the immaculately restored Pico House. Built in an Italianate style in 1870, it began life as a premier hotel and was the city's first three-story building.

More treasures beckon to the west of the plaza. **Cross Main to get to Our Lady Queen of Angels (La Placita) Catholic Church.** Dedicated in 1822, it's the oldest church in Los Angeles. Behind it is an ancient cemetery that includes a vertical cactus garden, which provides a surprisingly appealing—and potentially pain-inducing—tapestry of colors and textures.

After our whirlwind tours of Chinatown and Paseo De La Plaza, it's time to close out the triangle. **Retrace your steps back to Alameda and turn right.** In about 800 steps, you'll enter Little Tokyo. **Cross Temple Street and turn right. On your left, locate the parking lot through the hedges, and walk through the lot** to get to the Go For Broke Monument, which honors the 16,000 Japanese American soldiers who served our country during World War II. Scanning their names in the polished black rock, it's impossible to not be moved, especially when you consider how they were forced into camps by the very same government they were now defending with their lives.

Find the walkway to the south of the monument. It will take you past the Geffen Contemporary at MOCA and the Japanese American National Museum. **Turn right on 1st Street.** Note the brass placards in the sidewalk spelling out a timeline of major events in Japanese American life. **At the middle of the block—339 1st Street—take the crosswalk to the south side of the street. Find the driveway a couple paces to your left and head down it** to take in the majestic Koyasan Buddhist Temple.

Return to 1st, turn right, and then right again through the Japanese Village Plaza. The outdoor mall lets out at 2nd Street. **Turn right on 2nd and cross over to the northwest corner of 2nd and San Pedro Street, accessing a diago-**

nal street named after Ellison Shoji Onizuka. This astronaut was the first Japanese American to reach space aboard the Space Shuttle *Discovery*, which made his death in the *Challenger* explosion in 1986 all the more tragic. A replica of the Space Shuttle is on display halfway down the lane.

Onizuka Street lets out onto 1st. **Cross over to the west side of Los Angeles Street and proceed north to Arcadia Street. Turn left. When you reach Broadway, take the crosswalk and go up the sweep of stairs just to the right. Via another crosswalk, cross over to the west sidewalk of Hill Street.** Immediately in front of you, you'll find a massive stone relief depicting the raising of the American flag on this site on July 4, 1847. The Fort Moore Pioneer Memorial honors the troops who helped secure California from Mexico.

Proceed a few paces north and find the wall etching that recounts the history of California. Take a moment to really appreciate the artisanship. If a public

> **EXTRA STEPS**
>
> What if you built a mall and no one came? That's pretty much what happened to the generically named Los Angeles Mall, a forgotten subterranean strip of vacant storefronts and sparse restaurants that only come alive for weekday lunchers. Enter this early '70s anachronism from the northwest corner of Los Angeles and Temple Streets.

lic work of this nature were on display in a European city, it would be a prized landmark. In Los Angeles, it's just another neglected shrine more familiar to homeless people than any of the thousands of commuters who blow by it every day. For us walkers, at least, it's a fitting capper to our exploration of L.A.'s roots, and another reminder that the best treasures are found on foot.

From the memorial, proceed 1,400 steps up Hill and back through Chinatown to your point of origin.

3

THE ARTS DISTRICT

INDUSTRIAL CHIC

Who says art and commerce can't mix? This loop east of downtown explores L.A.'s industrial district— revitalized and reimagined as an artists' enclave— while crossing three of the Los Angeles River's fourteen historic bridges.

- **TERRAIN:** Flat with stairs
- **SURFACE:** Paved
- **FIDO FRIENDLY?:** Yes
- **PARKING:** Street parking on Mission Road, near 1st Street, Los Angeles

There was a time in the not-too-distant past when the region east of Central Avenue was a forgotten no man's land of empty brick factories and broken windows, a ready-made, post-apocalyptic backdrop for movies like *Repo Man*. It was a far cry from the early twentieth century, when a slew of wholesale industries—from foundry and furniture to rubber and apparel—set up shop here. Proximity to nearby railroad terminals ensured that goods could be moved quickly across the country.

As businesses moved their operations elsewhere, the infrastructure remained behind. Like hermit crabs clambering into spacious shells, creative types moved into the abandoned warehouses, establishing a toehold that has resulted in the still-evolving Arts District of today.

A walk through the Arts District starts with the ultimate welcome mat in the form of the 1st Street Viaduct. **Start on**

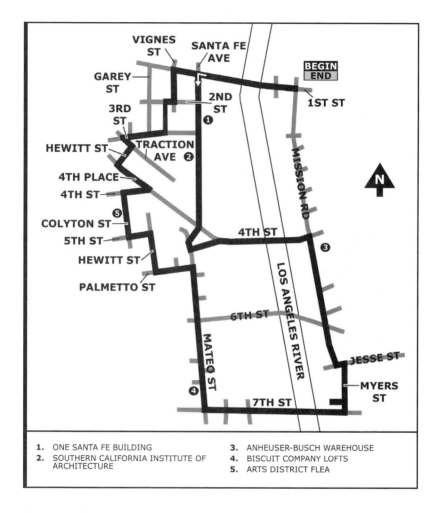

VIGNES ST
SANTA FE AVE
GAREY ST
BEGIN END
3RD ST
2ND ST
1ST ST
HEWITT ST
TRACTION AVE
4TH PLACE
4TH ST
COLYTON ST
5TH ST
HEWITT ST
PALMETTO ST
4TH ST
MISSION RD
LOS ANGELES RIVER
6TH ST
MATEO ST
JESSE ST
MYERS ST
7TH ST
N

1. ONE SANTA FE BUILDING
2. SOUTHERN CALIFORNIA INSTITUTE OF ARCHITECTURE
3. ANHEUSER-BUSCH WAREHOUSE
4. BISCUIT COMPANY LOFTS
5. ARTS DISTRICT FLEA

the southwest corner of 1st Street and Mission. As you **head west over the 1,300-foot bridge**—the downtown skyline seemingly sprouting from the ground—you'll come across the first of several cornice-topped arches with viewing platforms under decorative lamps. No, you're not in Paris, but Angelenos did have romanticized notions of bridges and rivers in the 1920s, back when a pre-straitjacketed L.A. River was our River Seine. As the city's Engineer of Bridges, Merrill Butler set about designing dozens of bridges that married

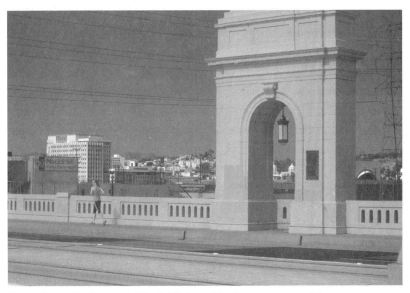

The 1st Street Bridge exemplifies L.A.'s beautification movement of the 1920s.

aesthetics and function. Almost 100 years later, his handiwork still makes the spirit soar.

About 600 steps into your journey, you'll come to a south-facing staircase, right where a giant sign stanchion bends over the roadway. **Take these steps down to Santa Fe Avenue.** The street marks the eastern edge of the Arts District and typifies the delicate dance between preserving the past and adjusting to the present. On your left is the One Santa Fe Building, a quarter-mile-long mixed-used complex with 430 units and 80,000 feet of retail space. On your right is the Southern California Institute of Architecture, housed in a former freight train depot. Note the boarded-up loading docks that run the length of the structure; they used to serve a track that ran down Santa Fe—named after the Santa Fe Southern Railway.

After 800 steps on Santa Fe, the avenue goes under the 4th Street Viaduct and turns eastward. **Look for the stairwell on the left side. Take it up to the viaduct and turn**

right. Heed the silent calls of those little concrete benches carved into the railing, imploring you

to sit and admire the views. Butler completed this bridge two years after its northern neighbor. But while the 1st Street Viaduct favors Classical elements, this one goes all Goth on us, with triangular interlaced rails and pitched archways instead of rounded ones.

As you approach the other side, find the southern stairwell just past the overhead steel sign. Take the steps down, turning left (south) onto Mission Road. This is an industrial artery with old and current railroad tracks bisecting the street—a reminder that the area east of the river is still very much factory-based. Just past the Anheuser-Busch warehouse, look for the weathered railroad crossing sign, one of the older railroad "X's" in Los Angeles.

After two blocks, Mission snakes under the 6th Street Viaduct. The original Merrill Butler bridge, built in 1932, had flying steel arches framing its Streamline Moderne truss. At 3,546 feet, it was once the longest concrete viaduct in the world. Unfortunately, the bridge's cement supports began to disintegrate due to a rare chemical reaction. The bridge is in the process of being replaced by a new one whose design combines past flourishes with modern safety features like bike lanes. A moment of silence, please, as we mourn the passing of the crown jewel of Merrill Butler's L.A. River viaducts. (I mean it—I'm watching you!)

Continue south on Mission. Hang a left on Jesse Street, then a quick right on Myers Street. Follow it for one block and turn right on Mission, which parallels the 7th Street Viaduct. Proceed on Mission for a few dozen steps to the parking lot fence that abuts the L.A. River. Turn your gaze toward the viaduct's span. Notice anything peculiar? It's a double-decker job. The bottom portion, supported by three arches, was erected in 1910 and used by streetcars. To save money, our man Merrill plopped a second level on top of it in 1929 to accommodate automobiles, entombing the trolley lanes underneath. It's inaccessible to all but the most hardened graffiti artists, urban spelunkers, and zombie hunters.

To cross the bridge, **walk back a few steps on Mission to the stairwell on the north side of it. Climb the steps and turn right.** The 7th Street Viaduct has the usual Butler hallmarks of sculpted railings and decorative lampposts.

Once on the other side, turn right on Mateo Street. On your left is a seven-story landmark that opened in 1925. *Chips Ahoy!*, Augustus Gloop, you have found the dream factory for Oreos and Mallomars! Yes, this was the headquarters for the National Biscuit Company, aka Nabisco. The building has since been converted to the Biscuit Company Lofts.

After several blocks, **turn left on Palmetto Street,** into the heart of the Arts District. Portions of Palmetto have a curb running right down the middle of the street, left over from train tracks that created two separate grades. Is the raised roadway supposed to accommodate eastbound cars? Or is it meant to be undriveable? Even motorists don't seem to know. But that's part of the fun of this district, making you want to enjoy its quirky charms before they're glossed over in the name of safety. Check out the brick edifice on your right from the early 1900s, also converted to lofts. As evidenced by the faded signage, it once headquartered the famous Barker Bros. furniture company, which

SIDE-STEP

After the new 6th Street Viaduct is complete, feel free to deviate from this walk while still keeping within 10,000 steps. Simply access the new bridge by turning left on 7th Street, left on Boyle Avenue, and left on Whittier Boulevard (which turns into 6th Street). Rejoin the book's route at Mateo Street. Or simply stick with the route below.

had a proud 111-year run in Los Angeles before folding in 1992.

Next, turn right on Hewitt Street. On the corner of Hewitt and 5th Street is an Urth Caffé, emerging like an oasis in the desolate cityscape. The place is always packed. If you can hold off a few more minutes, there are more meal options around the corner; otherwise, this is a prime spot for a delicious pastry or a refreshing smoothie.

Turn left on 5th, then right on Coylton Street, entering a block-long stretch with murals known as the Arts District Flea, a large indoor flea market. At the end of the block, **swing right on 4th Street, then make a hairpin turn onto 4th Place. Turn right on Hewitt, which takes you to Traction Avenue.** This is where all the hungry artists go. Take your pick from a number of eateries serving up burgers, gourmet sausages, or vegan fare. Don't forget to hit up the Pie Hole for a flaky dessert that's as exotic as its pierced patrons. My favorite: Earl Grey Tea Pie.

From Traction, turn right on 3rd Street. A few steps past Garey Street, turn left into an unmarked alleyway just to the west of a four-story brick building. (If you miss it, just take Garey Street.) The left side of the alley still has a rail line, its wall a canvas for ever-changing street art. The structure on the right used to be R23, a famous sushi joint. Corrugated awnings still hang over the former loading docks.

At the end of the alley, turn right on 2nd Street, left on Vignes Street, and right on 1st Street. Take 1st over the viaduct, back to your starting point in Boyle Heights.

Now thank yourself for supporting the arts.

4

BOYLE HEIGHTS / LINCOLN HEIGHTS

GATEWAY TO EAST— AND OLD—L.A.

Like uninvited guests at a party, three major freeways trample through Boyle and Lincoln Heights, slicing up key landmarks like Hollenbeck Park. But links to old L.A. and the region's Mexican heritage are still very much intact, if you know where to look.

- **TERRAIN:** Flat with slight inclines
- **SURFACE:** Mostly paved
- **FIDO FRIENDLY?:** Yes
- **PARKING:** Street parking near Mariachi Plaza, at Boyle Avenue and 1st Street, Boyle Heights

Boyle Heights: named after an Irishman, populated by Jews, now largely Latino. It's the true mutt community of Los Angeles, drawing a mix of immigrants over its 150-plus years. Andrew A. Boyle set the tone himself in 1858. Living harmoniously alongside American Indians and Mexicans, he was the first white Angeleno to live east of the Los Angeles River. He also built the first bridges into the city.

This walk starts in the spiritual heart of Boyle Heights— **Mariachi Plaza, located on the northeast corner of 1st Street and Boyle Avenue.** On any given day, especially weekends, it attracts dozens of charro-suited men. Some come with guitars slung over shoulders and trumpets in hand, others with nothing more than smiles and business cards—all hoping to be hired for a day's work of honest song.

It's been this way, on this corner, since the 1930s. The

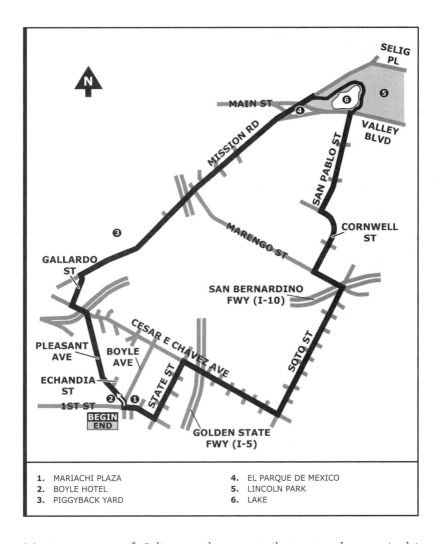

1. MARIACHI PLAZA
2. BOYLE HOTEL
3. PIGGYBACK YARD
4. EL PARQUE DE MEXICO
5. LINCOLN PARK
6. LAKE

Mexican state of Jalisco, a key contributor to the mariachi movement, donated the small pavilion for impromptu performances. The plaza also hosts a marketplace, public art, and an iconic bookstore known as Libros Schmibros—its very name a nod to Boyle Heights's dual heritage of Jews and Hispanics.

From Mariachi Plaza, cross over to the other side of Boyle. Gawk at the four-story Italianate apartment building. It dates to 1889, opening with much fanfare as the Boyle

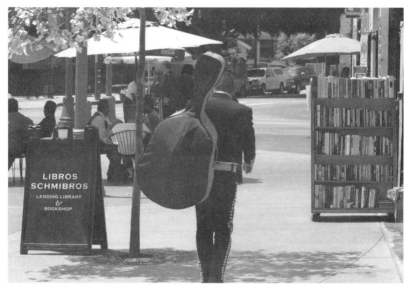

A charro-suited mariachi strolls through Mariachi Plaza, hefting his tools of the trade.

Hotel—the "Gateway to East Los Angeles." It eventually fell into disrepair before undergoing a recent $20 million facelift. From day one, the building was a magnet for mariachi players, earning the nickname the Mariachi Hotel. It now has a designated practice space for musicians.

Traipse a few paces north on Boyle, turning left on Pleasant Avenue. Though this street may appear anything but pleasant, look closer and spot the few clapboard homes that have managed to hold off the wrecking ball (or a horrible stucco makeover), like the Victorian at 1623, and two more near the corner of Echandia Street. To the west, off in the distance, is the San Antonio Winery, the last of eighty wineries once clustered near downtown before Prohibition. Mr. Boyle owned a vineyard

STEPPING BACK

In the late eighteenth century, the Pleasant Avenue region drew a wave of French Basque families, whose sheep grazed the hillside down to the untamed Los Angeles River below.

that ran along the eastern banks of the river. So *that's* why he built those bridges!

When you reach the T-intersection with Cesar E. Chavez Avenue, make a left, then a quick right on Gallardo Street, which runs into Mission Road. Turn right on Mission, entering Lincoln Heights. On your left is a sprawling trainyard known as Piggyback Yard, owned by Union Pacific Railroad for over 100 years. With its proximity to the L.A. River, downtown, Boyle Heights, and Lincoln Heights, future plans may include converting the 125-acre industrial plot into a verdant plateau of restored river habitat and mixed-use parkland.

Stay on Mission for 2,000 steps, then cross Valley Boulevard. On the right side, just past the bridge, is a statue of Mexican Revolution hero Pancho Villa on horseback. **A few steps past Pancho, enter the block-long El Parque de Mexico,** where you'll find a mission bell and two dozen statues of even more Mexican heroes (and heroines). Just east of the shrine is another statue of a Mexican revolutionary on horseback—Jose Maria Morelos. For good measure, El Parque de Mexico spills over to a green triangle north of Mission, where there are two *more* statues. All told, you'd be hard-pressed to find more outdoor sculptures per square foot in L.A. than you'll find in this de facto museum devoted to Mexican history.

Staying on Mission, go past Main Street and find the decomposed granite walking path into Lincoln Park. Hidden on your right is—you guessed it—another statue, this one of President Lincoln, arms folded, sternly guarding his namesake park. In the 1880s, Southern Pacific Railroad transferred this parcel of land to the city. By the early 1900s, Eastlake Park (as it was then called) had developed into a thriving amusement center, a counterpart to Westlake (now MacArthur) Park, which was considered the Westside of Los Angeles at the time.

Eastlake Park hosted the city's first zoo, owned by movie pioneer William Selig. Finding resi-

PICNIC OP

Lakeside at Lincoln Park, 3501 Valley Boulevard.

dents for the zoo was easy—he just donated wild animals that had appeared in his films. By 1915, the zoo had swelled to over 700 species. The old entrance to the zoo is at the corner of Mission and Selig Place. Where tigers once roamed, teenagers now kickflip at the Lincoln Park Skatepark.

One feature of the park that hasn't changed is its lake, built over a long-buried stream. Its brick boathouse still stands on the northern shore, a holdout from the park's recreational heyday. One can easily imagine bands playing show tunes here before an audience of mustachioed men and Victorian-garbed women, as boys in knickers ran off to check out the alligator farm and grandmas settled their tired bones into the hot sulphur springs. These days, the lake's biggest draw is its vociferous ducks, though you will find stubborn fishermen trying to lure catfish onto their hooks.

Exit the park by following the pathway along the lake's north and east shore toward Valley Boulevard. If you can stand to see one more statue, there is one of Florence Nightingale that was commissioned by the Works Progress Administration in 1937. Sadly, the Lady of the Lamp looks more like the *Venus de Milo*, her hands lost to the years.

Return to your starting point by taking a more direct path: crossing Valley Boulevard, head south on San Pablo Street. After passing a hospital and another park, turn left on Cornwell Street, left on Marengo Street, and right on Soto Street. On the southeast corner of Soto and Cesar Chavez is King Taco, an East L.A. institution whose owner sold tacos out of a converted ice cream truck before expanding into a mini-empire of over twenty restaurants. "Sava the flava" of their legendary hot sauce on your favorite Mexican dish. Or, for an equally authentic experience, **head**

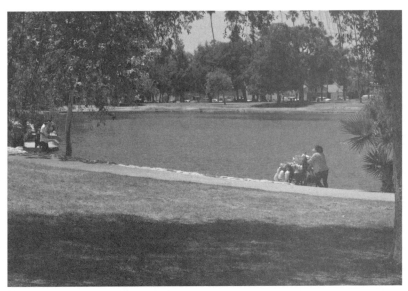

A lake dating to the 1890s forms the centerpiece of Lincoln Park.

three blocks west on Cesar Chavez to Guisados Tacos. The tacos come in a variety of marinated meats and veggies, served in homemade mini-tortillas. Can't decide? The sample platter has you covered.

From Guisados, it's 1,200 steps back to your car. Simply **take Cesar Chavez to State Street and make a left. Turn right on 1st Street, returning to Mariachi Plaza.** As you nod to the same mariachi players you saw before, you think, *y'know, it would be really cool to hire these guys to play at my next backyard barbecue.*

5

ECHO PARK / ANGELINO HEIGHTS

ECHOES OF DECADES PAST

Bookended by two extraordinary parks—whose origins are 150 years apart—this loop pays tribute to Echo Park's idiosyncratic past, with a detour to its classy neighbor, Angelino Heights.

- **TERRAIN:** Flat with slight inclines
- **SURFACE:** Mostly paved
- **FIDO FRIENDLY?:** Yes
- **PARKING:** Street parking near Angelus Temple at 1100 Glendale Boulevard, Echo Park

Echo Park has long drawn radical artists, free thinkers, and fiery gurus, a sort of Eastside answer to Venice Beach. By the 1920s, it was filled with so many communists, it was known as "Red Hill."

During that time, a colorful evangelist named Aimee Semple McPherson was the unofficial queen of Echo Park. **This walk starts at the historic Angelus Temple,** founded by McPherson in 1923. Parishioners regularly packed the 5,300 seats of her church, which at one time boasted the largest unsupported concrete dome in the nation. Aimee's flock extended well beyond Echo Park's borders, earning her a line in the song "Hooray for Hollywood" ("Aimee Semple" rhyming with "Shirley Temple").

From Angelus Temple, head south by crossing Park Avenue to Echo Park Lake, created way back in the 1860s as a man-made reservoir. If you ever want to know the current state of Los Angeles after being away for a while, a good place

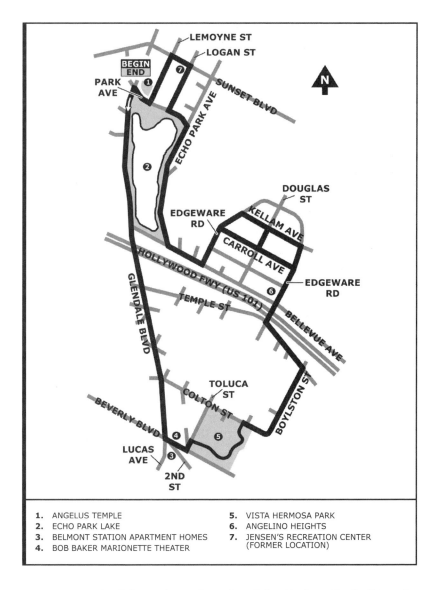

1. ANGELUS TEMPLE
2. ECHO PARK LAKE
3. BELMONT STATION APARTMENT HOMES
4. BOB BAKER MARIONETTE THEATER
5. VISTA HERMOSA PARK
6. ANGELINO HEIGHTS
7. JENSEN'S RECREATION CENTER
   (FORMER LOCATION)

to start are its lake-oriented parks (MacArthur Park, Lincoln Park, Echo Park, etc.). During the record crime of the early 1990s, this was not a place where you felt safe. But today, the twenty-nine-acre park is as much a home for picnicking Central American families as it is for millennials paddle-boating

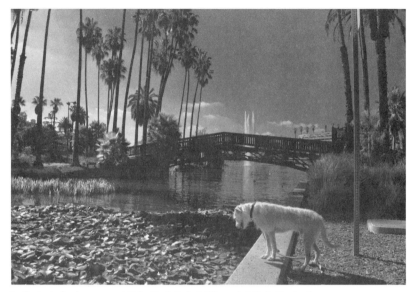

Is that a tadpole amongst Echo Park Lake's lily pads? Only Porter knows.

around the fountain or Silver Lake rockers doing photo shoots.

As you walk south, stay on the east side of Glendale.
Notice the lotus plants to the left, the centerpiece of the park's ever-popular annual Lotus Festival, celebrated every summer.

When you get to the southern end of the lake, continue under the Hollywood Freeway (US 101). Two thousand steps down Glendale, shaded by the Beverly Boulevard overpass, you'll come to a fork: Lucas Avenue to the right and 2nd Street to the left. At the

STEPPING BACK

Capitalizing on Echo Park's free-spirited ways, A. Victor Segno duped thousands of followers into joining his Segno Success Club in the early 1900s. In return for monthly fees, this brainiac claimed to send out brain waves to his followers that would guarantee them phenomenal success. He eventually built a gaudy temple called the American Institute of Mentalism on the cliff to your right, overlooking the lake. It was torn down in the 1960s, several decades after Segno himself vanished without a trace.

confluence of these streets—1304 2nd Street—is a modern residential building. A sign identifies it as the Belmont Station Apartment Homes, with a picture of a red streetcar. The train is a reminder that this site used to be a tunnel entrance for L.A.'s first subway, a full sixty-five years before the Blue Line ushered in a new era of subways that we now take for granted. The "Hollywood Subway," as it was incongruously called, only traveled one mile to the Subway Terminal Building downtown. But at its peak, 65,000 passengers made the trip daily. After the subway shut down in the '50s, the tunnel was still visible well into the 2000s, a favored spot for street artists until the apartment complex went up.

Stay on the Glendale sidewalk until it curves eastward, past the site of the old Bob Baker Marionette Theater. Cross over to the east side of Toluca Street. On your right you'll see a sign and parking lot for Vista Hermosa Park. Enter the park grounds and find the walking trail that takes you to its higher reaches.

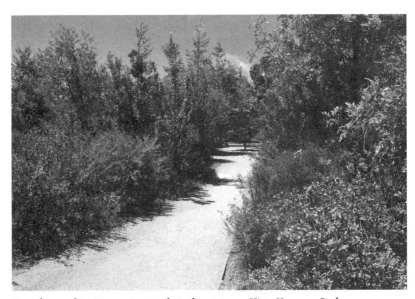

One of several inviting nature trails in the 10.5-acre Vista Hermosa Park.

While Echo Park Lake is one of the oldest parks in the city, Vista Hermosa is one of the newest. As such, it has an eco-friendly, quasi-wild vibe that encourages exploration. Winding pathways glide past waterfalls and streams flowing through meadows and native trees. And did I mention the downtown skyline is the backdrop to it all? You'll easily burn off 1,200 steps loafing about this tucked-away treasure. By the time you leave the park, you'll be at 4,000 steps.

Exit at the northern gate along Colton Street. Make a right on Colton, which curves and heads north as Boylston Street. Turn left at Temple Street. The next three blocks of Temple—from Boylston to Edgeware Road—are fairly nondescript. Not so in 1886. Less than ten years after the debut of the cable car in San Francisco, this section marked the beginning of L.A.'s own cable car line, which extended all the way to Main Street. It lasted until 1902, when Henry Huntington bought and converted the line to electric streetcars.

Upon reaching Edgeware, make a right. Pass over the Hollywood Freeway and Bellevue Avenue, entering the old Victorian neighborhood known as Angelino Heights (some signs say "Angeleno Heights"). Mere steps from Temple's former cable cars, this is where the city's elite settled in the 1880s.

Turn left on Carroll Avenue—a National Register Historic District—and gape at the magnificently restored homes from the late nineteenth century. While Carroll holds the cream of the crop, you can find other Queen Anne Victorians and California bungalows on adjacent streets like Douglas Street and Kellam Avenue.

After you've sufficiently absorbed L.A.'s first true suburb, **head back down to Bellevue, which you can access via Edgeware or Douglas. Turn right on Bellevue and cross Echo Park Avenue.** You will end up

PICNIC OP
Northern shore of Echo Park Lake, near Park Avenue.

on the east shoreline of Echo Park Lake. **Turn right onto the walkway.** Halfway up is the restored boathouse, which rents paddleboats. Take a load off and grab a bite or a beverage at the boathouse's restaurant.

From the boathouse, continue up Echo Park Avenue's sidewalk. Turn left on Park Avenue. Admire the enchanting "Queen of the Angels" statue at the north end of the lake. Also known as the "Lady of the Lake," she was designed by female sculptor Ada May Sharpless during the New Deal era.

From Park, take Logan Street to Sunset Boulevard. On the southwest corner of Logan and Sunset is an Italian Romanesque, mixed-use building—one of L.A.'s first—from 1924. The Historic-Cultural Monument sports a seventeen-by-twenty-eight-foot rooftop sign (best seen from across the street). It reads "Jensen's Recreation Center," and shows a man bowling, with 1,300 multicolored light bulbs that predate L.A.'s neon sign craze. After being dark for fifty years, the sign flickered back to life in 1997, though the actual bowling alley it advertises is long gone.

Turn left onto Lemoyne Street. It's a quick jaunt back to your point of departure—the Angelus Temple. Ms. McPherson, who was known for her revivals, must surely be smiling somewhere about Echo Park's.

6

ELYSIAN PARK WEST

TREASURES LOST AND FOUND

The next time someone accuses L.A. of lacking in history, tell them to take a hike. Better yet, take them on this one, where you encounter five landmarks that are at least ninety years old.

- ■ **TERRAIN:** Flat with stairs and slight inclines
- ■ **SURFACE:** Mostly paved
- ■ **FIDO FRIENDLY?:** Yes
- ■ **PARKING:** Lot adjacent to Grace E. Simons Lodge, at 1025 Elysian Park Drive, Los Angeles

The Eastside of Los Angeles is anchored by its two biggest parks—Griffith and Elysian. If these parks were siblings, Elysian would forever live in her big sis's shadow. Where Griffith Park wears her charms on the surface, Elysian Park has to earn your adoration. But once she does, L.A.'s oldest park rewards you with some of the city's most beguiling lost treasures.

Start your walk from the parking lot for the Grace E. Simons Lodge. Access the slightly obscured trailhead to the left of the lodge's black, wrought-iron gate. The first thing you'll notice are boney trees drooping over an unmaintained nature trail that zigzags through graffiti-laden rocks. Ladies and gentlemen, I give you the Elysian Park Arboretum! Yes, unfortunately, age and neglect have caught up with L.A.'s first arboretum. Founded in 1893, it once boasted 140 species of trees from around the world. Still, hints of its past

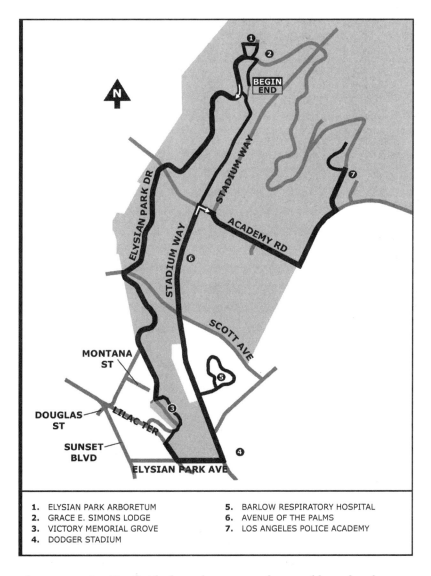

1. ELYSIAN PARK ARBORETUM
2. GRACE E. SIMONS LODGE
3. VICTORY MEMORIAL GROVE
4. DODGER STADIUM
5. BARLOW RESPIRATORY HOSPITAL
6. AVENUE OF THE PALMS
7. LOS ANGELES POLICE ACADEMY

glory remain. Trailside benches carved out of logs beckon to your bottom. Placards give up the trees' secrets ("California Buckeye: *Aesculus californica*. Nuts used for food after leaching, leaves & nuts used to stun fish"). Other facts are not quite so fascinating ("Wood grows as trees get older. Wood is great building material"). To that, I say: "Air. We breathe it."

After exploring this shaggy-dog sanctuary, **trek a couple hundred steps east to the western fence of the Grace E. Simons Lodge.** Simons was an Elysian Park preservationist who worked for the *California Eagle* newspaper, where she earned the respect of Malcolm X for her tough reporting style. Spy on the lodge's "backyard," which can be rented out for weddings and special events. Envy its storybook pathways and bridges over a babbling man-made brook as you ponder the impossibly blue water straight out of a Technicolor musical. Most of all, consider how this perfectly coiffed garden lies in such stark contrast to the pining trees you just came from. (If you want to walk this garden, a side gate near the front entrance is often open on weekdays.)

With 1,000 steps under your belt—or your feet—**access Elysian Park Drive, just west of the parking lot.** The street, which divides Echo Park from Elysian Park, is closed to vehicles for the next 3,000 steps, making it a popular route for dog-walkers and bicyclists. Check out the sweeping views

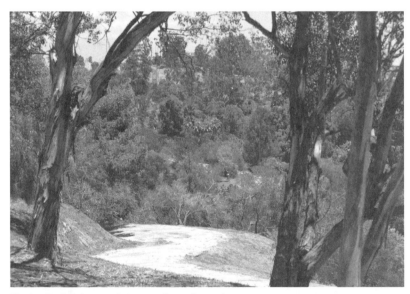

Elysian Park Drive wends its way through eucalyptus trees.

of Dodger Stadium and the Avenue of the Palms to your left. Picture yourself bushwhacking this path alongside Gaspar de Portolà, the Spanish explorer who trod these same grounds in 1769 on his way to claiming Alta California for Spain.

EXTRA STEPS

If you're looking to fill your belly, Sunset Boulevard is just two blocks away—one block down Montana Street, another block down Douglas Street. Two of the closest restaurants are The Park (1400 Sunset), which offers delectable upscale fare, and El Compadre (1449 Sunset), whose Mexi-gringo grub goes great with a flaming margarita!

Just past the cul-de-sac for Montana Street, you'll encounter ten steps on your left. They lead to a parcel of dirt that is actually part of the nearly 100-year-old Victory Memorial Grove, yet another forgotten Elysian Park landmark. Its most prominent feature is a bronze plaque on a boulder commemorating local fallen heroes of World War I. Erected by the Daughters of the American Revolution in 1921, its inscriptions of names and ranks below an engraved eagle are chill-inducing. As with the arboretum, the once-thriving forest of trees that were planted by the families of servicemen are now mostly reduced to a small army of steadfast eucalyptus.

From the memorial, it's another 1,000 steps to your next destination. **Follow the concrete walkway that parallels Elysian Park Drive to that street's hairpin turn. Cut across a green median to Lilac Terrace. Turn left, then left again on Elysian Park Avenue.** In front of you are signs for Dodger Stadium. Banish your thoughts of Dodger Dogs (they're overrated anyway). **Turn left on Stadium Way, and proceed 300 steps down the street to locate the cluster of cottages on your right.** These make up the Barlow Respiratory Hospital,

PICNIC OP

Elysian Park, near the "Avenue of the Palms" at Stadium Way, between Academy Road and Scott Avenue.

a long-term facility that started as a tuberculosis sanatorium in the early 1900s. Because sunlight and dry air were deemed the best balms for TB patients, it was designed with an eye toward getting patients outside to wander its twenty-five acres.

Wander onto the property, and scavenger-hunt for antiquities: boarded-up wood cabins that seem straight out of a kids-camp horror flick; a stone sundial near the library, dated 1902; decades-old citrus trees; and even a rusted-out chicken coop shaded by an ancient oak. Plans are underway to modernize this whole area (a quaint gift shop in a former dormitory shuttered mere weeks after I visited it), so hopefully you can experience these frozen-in-amber curios before the bulldozers move in.

After an 800-step amble through Barlow, **continue north on Stadium Way.** Just past Scott Avenue, you will stride through the nicknamed Avenue of the Palms. Its two rows of Canary Island Palms were planted in 1895. Sadly, disease and age have taken their toll, and plans are in motion to replace them. As with Barlow Hospital's original grounds, enjoy these beauts while you still can.

Next, make a right at Academy Road, heading toward another entrance to Dodger Stadium. Just before you hit the stadium's parking booths, Academy will jog to the left and take you to the entrance of the Los Angeles Police Academy, which has been training and swearing in officers since the 1920s. Its old-school restaurant is open to the public during weekdays, offering another lunch option. After admiring the café's firearm collection, visit the waterfall-laden rock garden in the back, trying to reconcile the incongruity of this little slice of paradise against the volley of gunfire from a nearby practice range.

From the Police Academy, it's 2,000 easy steps back to your car. **Double back on Academy Road and turn right into the parking lot just past Stadium Way.** At the end of the lot is a narrow walking path that parallels Stadium Way. **Take the**

path all the way back to the Grace E. Simons lot.

Congratulations! You have found the lost riches of L.A.'s oldest park, and you still haven't even covered its eastern portion. Who's ready for a sequel . . . ?

7

ELYSIAN PARK EAST

BETWEEN A ROCK AND A FREEWAY

Ever wondered what it's like to walk on a freeway? This intrepid urban trek takes you as close as you can safely get, depositing you in the quiet of Elysian Park and a mysterious hilltop garden.

■ **TERRAIN:** Flat with stairs and moderate inclines
■ **SURFACE:** Mostly paved
■ **FIDO FRIENDLY?:** Yes
■ **PARKING:** Street parking on Avenue 28, near Figueroa Street, Los Angeles

For better or for worse, freeways define Los Angeles. At one point in the 1950s, dozens were planned that would've ripped the heart and soul out of places like Beverly Hills, Laurel Canyon, and South Pasadena. Fortunately, most of these projects never came to fruition, but neighborhoods like Whitley Heights and South L.A. weren't so lucky. Elysian Park falls into this latter camp. The city's most celebrated early freeway, the Arroyo Seco Parkway (SR 110), sliced through the eastern section of L.A.'s oldest park. Not to worry, dear walkers. To ensure public access to the park (and to prove that even traffic engineers have a sense of humor) the Elysian Park portion of freeway was built with a sidewalk that allows pedestrians to walk alongside it.

From the intersection of Avenue 28 and Figueroa Street, walk south on Figueroa, passing multiple restaurants. If you feel like sitting down for a meal, now's your only

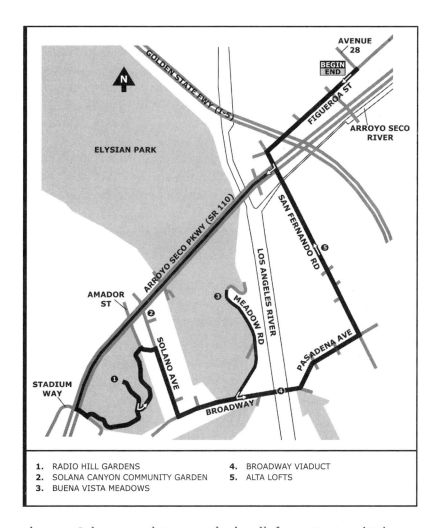

1. RADIO HILL GARDENS
2. SOLANA CANYON COMMUNITY GARDEN
3. BUENA VISTA MEADOWS
4. BROADWAY VIADUCT
5. ALTA LOFTS

chance. Otherwise, this is an ideal walk for a picnic, which you can enjoy in Elysian Park.

After passing under the Golden State Freeway (I-5), you'll come to the next cross-street, San Fernando Road—once part of historic Route 99. **Turn left on San Fernando, staying on the north sidewalk. A couple dozen steps later, pass under the southbound lanes of the Arroyo Seco Parkway. Stop short of the northbound lanes, and find the break in the wall to your left, which leads to a seemingly**

forgotten stairway. Climb the steps. You'll land between the north- and southbound lanes of the freeway.

    Hook a U-turn at the top of the stairs, and head south. You will suddenly find yourself smack dab in the middle of the freeway. Two questions immediately come to mind: Am I allowed to be here? (Yes.) And whoever thought this was a good idea? (I dunno . . . the same kind of masterminds who approved the Green Line bypassing LAX?) Being hemmed in by six lanes of rushing traffic is as unnerving as a Magic Mountain rollercoaster, but you can take some measure of comfort in the barricaded fence that keeps you from ending up as roadkill.

    After about 200 steps, you'll pass over the Metro Gold Line tracks and the confluence where the Arroyo Seco and Los Angeles River come together. To your left, the first of four Figueroa tunnels will come into view. Before the freeway was built, Figueroa's north- and southbound lanes utilized these tunnels. Now, the tunnels carry northbound traffic for the 110. The freeway's tunnel-less southbound lanes—which you'll be paralleling from this point on—extend just to the west at a higher grade.

    Which brings us to the next staircase. Not just any staircase, but a spiral staircase straight out of a Berliner's postwar urban dreamscape. You may have seen these mysterious steps a thousand times when driving the I-5 North transition out of the tunnels. I'm not much of a ghost guy, but every time I drive by these swirling steps, it seems like the perfect place to spot a Specter of the Freeways lording over late-night traffic, its black trench coat billowing in ashen clouds of exhaust.

    Turns out, these steps are simply a continuation of the walkway you're currently on. **Wind upwards on the staircase,** and you will find yourself flush against the fast lane of the southbound lanes to your right, with the granite face of Elysian Park to your left.

    Continue on this freeway-adjacent walkway. You will

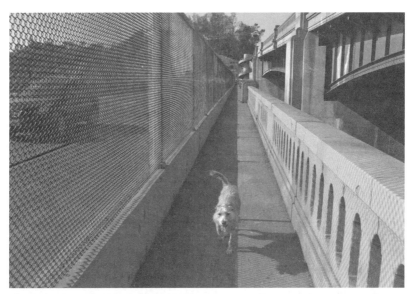

This is the closest you (or your dog) will ever get to walking on a freeway. Note the spiral staircase in the background.

see occasional openings in the fence that lead to trails into the chaparral. Admire the old-time decorative lampposts and Art Deco details of the tunnels.

About 2,000 steps from your starting point, the walkway will switchback down a ramp, dumping you onto Stadium Way. **Take this walkway, then turn left, crossing over the northbound freeway lanes.** Just past the bridge, two trails will come into view on the left—a dirt path and an unmarked paved road closed to vehicles. **Choose the paved road,** whose gentle incline offers an impressive view of L.A.'s steel-and-concrete skyline east of the river.

As the road begins to curve northward, you'll come to a fork. Make a left, which will take you to Radio Hill Gardens. Like the Elysian Park Arboretum in our other Elysian Park walk, this is one of those public parks that the city seems to have consigned to oblivion. I've yet to see another soul at this place, a sad patch of browning foliage amidst fogged-over kiosks, turned-over benches, and nonfunctioning water fountains—not so much deferred maintenance as deterred maintenance. Presiding over it all is a telecommunications tower that lends the park its name. Maybe if they added a Starbucks here, things would pick up . . . ? **Head back down the way you came, reconnecting with the main paved road. Turn left and follow it to Amador Street,** watching for the reappearance

EXTRA STEPS

One block north of the intersection of Amador Street and Solano Avenue is the Solano Canyon Community Garden. The fact that it's flush against the northbound lanes of the 110 is not a coincidence. The garden is located on the former site of Solano Avenue Elementary School, which was torn down in 1935 to make room for the freeway. The garden's orchard actually extends over the tunnel that lies just to the north.

PICNIC OP

Buena Vista Meadows Picnic Area, near the end of Meadow Road.

of cars. **Make a right on Amador, then walk a few short steps to Solano Avenue.** A "Little Free Library" sits on the corner, with a sign encouraging the exchange of books, seeds, or recipes. It looks like a wooden birdfeeder with a door. Just another example of the little finds waiting to be found when you take to the streets of L.A.

Turn right on Solano, then left on Broadway. After 400 steps—just before the bridge—turn left onto Meadow Road, Elysian Park's eastern entrance. Stay on this road (ignoring the smaller road that forks off to the left) until you get to Buena Vista Meadows, an underserved, hidden oasis. **Return to Broadway by simply doubling back.**

After turning left on Broadway, proceed over the Broadway Viaduct, a 1911 Beaux-Arts masterpiece with twelve viewing balconies and two pairs of fluted Ionic columns topped by intricate cornices. **Make a left on Pasadena Avenue, then another left on San Fernando Road.**

Many of the buildings in this highly industrial area are being converted to lofts. My favorite: the Alta Lofts at 342 San Fernando, housed in a 1925 edifice that once served as the headquarters for Goodwill Industries. Note the streamlined signage that betrays the WPA's handiwork.

Continue on San Fernando for 600 steps, then turn right on Figueroa. In a few blocks you'll be back where you started, ending a walk in the park that was no ordinary walk in the park.

8

HIGHLAND PARK / MOUNT WASHINGTON

HOUSES OF THE HOLY

With an emphasis on historic homes, this walk visits eight Highland Park houses awarded protected status before chugging up a former railway route to the grandest—and most sacred—monument of them all atop Mount Washington.

- **TERRAIN:** Flat with stairs and one long, steep incline
- **SURFACE:** Mostly paved
- **FIDO FRIENDLY?:** No (not allowed on the Self-Realization Fellowship premises)
- **PARKING:** Street parking near the intersection of Carlota Boulevard and Avenue 43, Highland Park

Flanked by hills along the Arroyo Seco, Highland Park was one of L.A.'s first suburbs, reachable from downtown via streetcar as early as 1894. Its location enticed audacious architects who used rocks from the arroyo as construction materials. Following a script sadly familiar to other Eastside communities, Highland Park eventually fell on hard times. But the very things that drew residents here over 100 years ago are now drawing them back—proximity to downtown, interesting architecture and culture, and access to parks and nature. In fact, its biggest challenge nowadays seems to be how to stem the inexorable tide of gentrification and prevent it from becoming, as locals derisively sneer, "another Silver Lake."

Fortunately, Highland Park's bones are very well-preserved. **From the southwest corner of Avenue 43 and**

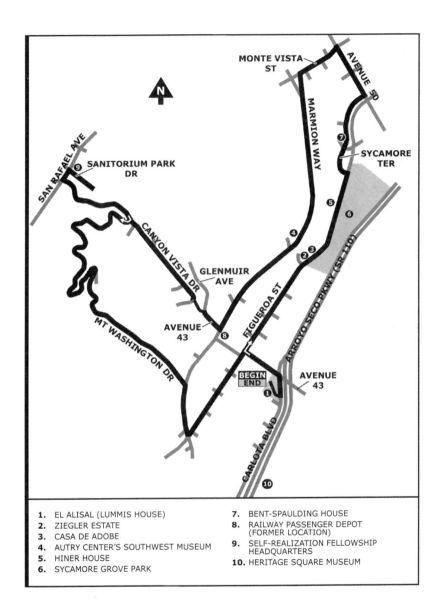

Legend:

1. EL ALISAL (LUMMIS HOUSE)
2. ZIEGLER ESTATE
3. CASA DE ADOBE
4. AUTRY CENTER'S SOUTHWEST MUSEUM
5. HINER HOUSE
6. SYCAMORE GROVE PARK
7. BENT-SPAULDING HOUSE
8. RAILWAY PASSENGER DEPOT (FORMER LOCATION)
9. SELF-REALIZATION FELLOWSHIP HEADQUARTERS
10. HERITAGE SQUARE MUSEUM

Carlota Boulevard, head a few paces down Carlota and enter the public grounds of El Alisal, more commonly known as the Lummis House. Take the pathway through the native-plant garden. Like a scene out of a fairy tale, the trees part to reveal the abode's stunning stone façade. It was built

by Charles Fletcher Lum-
mis between 1896 and
1910. That might seem
like a long time until you
learn that the American
Indian rights advocate
pretty much did every-
thing himself. Observe

STEPPING BACK

Charles Fletcher Lummis also
founded the Southwest Museum
in 1907. It moved to its Mount
Washington location in 1914.
Lummis was also an avid walker,
once walking from Cincinnati to
Los Angeles—4,200,000 steps!

the bell embedded in the mission-style "rock-itecture." (Don't
even try to trademark that term—I hereby bequeath it to public domain.) The inside is equally impressive, with exposed
wooden cross-beams and handcrafted furniture, an amalgam
of English Arts and Crafts and Pueblo Indian. For good measure, there's also a lily pond out back.

**After traversing the grounds, exit the Lummis House
the way you came in. Head north on Carlota, then left
on Avenue 43. When you reach Figueroa Street, cross
over to the other side and turn right.** Figueroa is one
of the longest and most storied streets in Los Angeles. It's
named after a governor of Alta California during Mexican
rule, though I'd like to start a petition to bring back its original name—Calle de los Chapules ("Grasshopper Street").
Who's with me?

About four blocks up Figueroa, look for the Ziegler Estate at 4601. The Victorian building—now a preschool—was
built in 1904. Next to it is Casa de Adobe, a 100-year-old hacienda built by the Hispanic Society of California with an
eye toward a more romantic bygone era. It's now owned by
the Autry Center's Southwest Museum, whose turreted tower
can be glimpsed on the hillside behind it. Just past Casa de
Adobe, at 4671, note the uphill staircase under a mission-style
archway splashed with a colorful mural. Like so many old L.A.
enclaves, the steps fed a trolley station, back when the Pacific
Electric Red Car rumbled through Highland Park.

Two hundred steps past the Red Car steps is the Hiner

House (4757 Figueroa), which blends into dense foliage. Built in 1922, it's a true architectural mongrel—a mix of Stone Tudor and California Chalet with Oriental accents—reflecting the anything-goes style of California. Its owner was a band leader who, when he wasn't playing concerts

EXTRA STEPS

Eight hundred steps from the Lummis Home is the Heritage Square Museum (at 3800 Homer Street). The price of admission gives you access to eight historic homes from the Victorian era and an old-time pharmacy, where tens of thousands of snake oil potions and magic health pills (Hazel's Wonder Tablets, anyone?) are on display.

across the street at Sycamore Grove Park, gave performances at the White House for President McKinley.

Walk another 200 steps and you will find yourself at the entrance of Sycamore Terrace, a short street that's long on history. In the 1890s, it was nicknamed "Professor's Row" due to all the faculty members from the original Occidental College who lived in its bungalows. The oldest is a Victorian/Craftsman hybrid at 4925 Sycamore Terrace known as the Bent-Spaulding House. Keep an eye out for other terrific examples of turn-of-the-century homes. Some of the more notable are at 4967, 4973, and 4985. (The Los Angeles Conservancy offers occasional interior tours of many Highland Park houses.) The residence at 4973 is perhaps the most unique, designed by the same architectural firm that built Hollywood's Chinese Theatre. Notice any similarities?

Walk to the end of Sycamore Terrace, which terminates at Avenue 50. On the corner you'll see Chico's, a divey Mexican restaurant that's become a local favorite. Enough culture for now—you're ready for the simple pleasures of killer potato tacos, shrimp burritos, and cinnamon coffee.

Properly recharged, you are now ready for loftier ambitions. **Go two blocks north on Avenue 50, then left on Monte Vista Street. After two and a half blocks, turn**

left on Marmion Way. Stay on Marmion for 1,800 steps, until you return to Avenue 43. Starting in 1909, a railway incline used to whisk people up Avenue 43 for a nickel. The train's destination was the burgeoning community of Mount Washington. From the corner of Avenue 43 and Marmion, you can spot the former Mission-style passenger depot across the Gold Line tracks.

To follow the path of the old railway, head up Avenue 43, which becomes Glenmuir Avenue after one block. Just as Glenmuir starts to turn right, locate the old stairway on the left side of the road and ascend the steps. They will connect you with Canyon Vista Drive. **After 700 steps, stay right at the fork** as Canyon Vista runs straight into Mount Washington Drive. It's another 700 steps to the apex at a fairly steep grade. Not to worry—you're about to be rewarded for your efforts!

Turn right on San Rafael Avenue. Two hundred feet later, turn right into a driveway known as Sanitorium Park Drive. A hilltop utopia unfurls before you in the footprint of the former Mount Washington Hotel. Served by the railway, it was the height of California chic in the 1910s. Charlie Chaplin and other moviemakers used to unwind up here after filming silents in Highland Park. Alas, the resort and the railway lost favor by the early '20s. The hotel was sold to Paramahansa Yogananda, a monk from the Swami Order of India and founder of the Self-Realization Fellowship. He lived and taught here for years, and it remains the world headquarters for the pan-religious organization. (Flip to the Pacific Palisades walk for a visit to the Self-Realization's Lake Shrine location.)

To see the grounds, **chug past the lawn to your right and down to the resort's former tennis courts,** which offer striking snapshots of downtown and beyond. Check out the sundial by the edge of the tennis courts. An inscription dates it to 1925, dedicated by the swami to his students.

From there, **take the gravel path** to the grove known

as the Temple of Leaves. Seek out a nice nook near the trickling stream. Find a hidden bench. Sit. Breathe. Silence your

PICNIC OP

Self-Realization Fellowship grounds, at 3880 San Rafael Avenue.

brain. I agree, it's terrifying. When you're ready, **continue on the pathway** until you get to a table and chairs carved out of stone. You think it looks like a prop out of *The Flintstones* movie. You've officially snapped back into the real world.

Continue up the path until you get to the paved parking area. Head along the driveway toward the exit. On your right is the edifice of the former hotel, now the headquarters for the fellowship. You'll also see a visitors center on your right before you leave the grounds.

Head back the way you came, making a left on San Rafael, then another left on Mount Washington Drive. Halfway down the hill, Mount Washington Drive makes a sharp hairpin turn to the right alongside a white fence. **Take this route, avoiding Canyon Vista (the street you came up).** After the railway shut down in 1921, Mount Washington Drive was the only way up the mountain. This is a wonderfully windy road surrounded by unexpected wilderness for its first 1,200 steps—a product of 1920s engineering, when roads conformed to the terrain of hillsides instead of just blasting through them. Stay vigilant of street signs as you reenter the residential area. Note the amazing old homes, with their odd-shaped lots and rock walls, that encapsulate the rugged appeal of Highland Park.

Continue on Mount Washington all the way down to Marmion. Turn right on Marmion, then left onto Figueroa. Four blocks later, make a right on Avenue 43, heading back to your car and the creature comforts of a material world.

9

SILVER LAKE

WALKING WITH SIR WALTER SCOTT

Forget its Flea-bitten Sunset Boulevard corridor. This crooked figure-eight walk connecting three reservoirs will have you believing that fairy tales do exist in Silver Lake. Or is it Silver Loch?

- **TERRAIN:** Flat with several slight inclines
- **SURFACE:** Mostly paved
- **FIDO FRIENDLY?:** Yes
- **PARKING:** Street parking near the Silver Lake Recreation Center, at 1850 Silver Lake Drive, Silver Lake

L et us commence with a eulogy for Los Angeles neighborhoods whose names are no longer with us: Owensmouth (now Canoga Park); Sherman (now West Hollywood); Edendale (now parts of Silver Lake and Echo Park) . . . the list goes on, but none were as whimsical as Ivanhoe.

Before the Silver Lake Reservoir was built in 1907, a Scottish developer named Hugo Reid took one look at the rolling green braes of present-day Silver Lake and thought of his native Scotland. He named the area after the famous novel by Sir Walter Scott, then dreamed up streets after characters in the book or names in his homeland—Saint George, Kenilworth, and Ben Lomond among them. Medieval Scotland is far removed from the boho-hipster hangout that Silver Lake has become, but the sense of whimsy remains in its hilly residential quarters, with a dip of the toe into Los Feliz.

Start at the Silver Lake Recreation Center, a neigh-

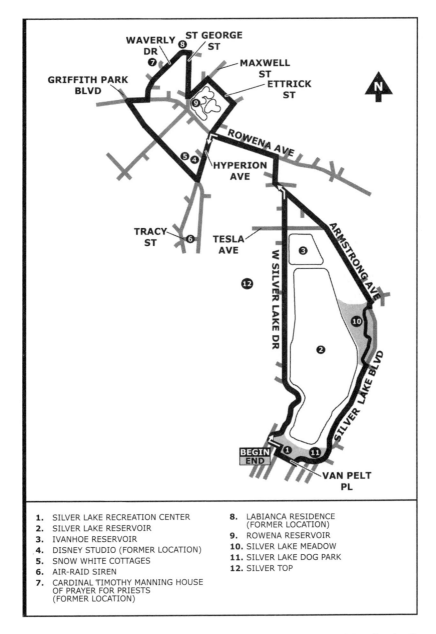

1. SILVER LAKE RECREATION CENTER
2. SILVER LAKE RESERVOIR
3. IVANHOE RESERVOIR
4. DISNEY STUDIO (FORMER LOCATION)
5. SNOW WHITE COTTAGES
6. AIR-RAID SIREN
7. CARDINAL TIMOTHY MANNING HOUSE
   OF PRAYER FOR PRIESTS
   (FORMER LOCATION)

8. LABIANCA RESIDENCE
   (FORMER LOCATION)
9. ROWENA RESERVOIR
10. SILVER LAKE MEADOW
11. SILVER LAKE DOG PARK
12. SILVER TOP

borhood park with a gymnasium, playground, and basketball courts. **Head north along the western shoreline of Silver Lake Reservoir (W. Silver Lake Drive),** part of a popular

2.2-mile loop. Though all three of the reservoirs on this walk once provided water to Eastside Angelenos, they have since been taken offline, replaced by the underground Headworks tanks near Griffith Park's Travel Town.

As you round the corner of the lake's dam, the sidewalk will turn into a dirt pathway. Through the fence on your right, you'll get your first view of the shimmering, 795-million-gallon Silver Lake Reservoir, which, at first glance, seems an apt name. On overcast days, the water has a silvery gray glow, reflecting the drab blacktop that lines its banks. In actuality, though, it's named after Herman Silver, a former water commissioner.

Sixteen hundred steps into your walk, the reservoir ends at a spillway that separates it from its little bro—Ivanhoe Reservoir. At the corner of Silver Lake Drive and Tesla Avenue, most pedestrians continue to the right and finish the loop. You, however, will **continue straight on Silver Lake Drive until it jogs left at Armstrong Avenue**—the 2,000-step mark. Follow the sidewalk another 400 steps and **make a left**

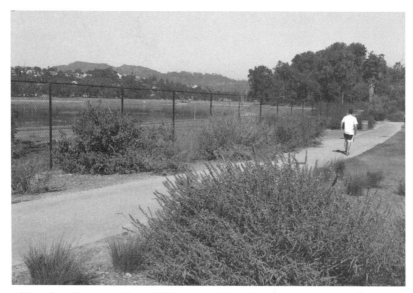

A lakeside pathway cuts through Silver Lake Meadow.

on Rowena Avenue—named, of course, after Ivanhoe's love interest. Across the street, the noble Saxon's spirit watches over his fair lady's namesake road from Ivanhoe Elementary. Founded in 1889, it's one of L.A.'s oldest public schools.

Continue on Rowena until you get to Hyperion Avenue. Cross the street and turn left, passing the supermarket to your right at 2719 Hyperion. It is here, from 1926 to 1940, that a young animator named Walt Disney ran his first legitimate studio, giving rise to a very famous rodent and the world's first feature-length cartoon, *Snow White and the Seven Dwarfs.* Look for the placard commemorating the studio on a lamppost on Hyperion, which in itself inspired the name of a theater at Disney California Adventure. Inside, near the cashiers, the grocery store displays an old photo of the studio.

Hang a right at the corner onto Griffith Park Boulevard. Behind the former Disney Studio are fairy-tale-style houses that resemble the cottage in the movie that the seven dwarfs live in. Disney lore says the *Snow White* animators took their inspiration for the dwarfs' dwelling from these 1931 bungalows. Indeed, director Hamilton Luske and several cartoonists occupied these bungalows at one time. The Norman Tower only adds to the medieval theme of this walk. Of course, David Lynch sees things through a darker prism, and staged a disturbing scene from his movie *Mulholland Drive* here.

EXTRA STEPS

Like many Angelenos who came of age during the Cold War, my childhood was haunted by the shrill scream of air-raid sirens, which were tested twelve times a year (the last Friday of every month at 10 AM). Many of the city's original 225 sirens are still standing, including a really rare one in the "birdhouse" design with a pleated platform that resembles a giant lampshade. It's 600 steps west of the corner of Hyperion and Griffith Park on Tracy Street, between the two aforementioned streets. Keep your eyes open for other sirens on these walks!

Push on up Griffith Park until you reconnect with Rowena Avenue. Make a right, then a quick left onto Waverly Drive. On your left, you'll find a stucco wall fronting a sprawling 8.5-acre estate whose grounds include—what else?—a mock medieval Renaissance castle. Initially inhabited by an L.A. radio tycoon, for decades the complex served as the Cardinal Timothy Manning House of Prayer for Priests, a silent retreat funded by the Archdiocese of Los Angeles.

Eerily, next door at 3311 Waverly (formerly 3301) stands a house with a long driveway behind a gate. On August 10, 1969, its occupants, Rosemary and Leno LaBianca, were butchered by the Manson Family, just one day after the even-more infamous murders at the Sharon Tate house on Benedict Canyon. While both killings were ordered by Charles Manson, he actually only set foot in this house before leaving his disciples to do the dirty work.

Now head south on Saint George Street for one block. Cross over to the other side of Maxwell Street and make a left. On your right is the block-long Rowena Reservoir. Gaze through the wrought-iron fence. Envy the lush landscape of orderly walking trails, trickling waterfalls, and little islands hosting preening waterfowl. Like artwork in a museum, you can look but you cannot touch . . . unless you work for the Department of Water and Power.

Turn right on Ettrick Street. After one block, take a right on Hyperion, then a left on Rowena. Retrace your steps to Silver Lake Reservoir, but this time continue straight on Armstrong Avenue instead of making a right on Silver Lake Drive. After 1,000 steps, turn right on Silver Lake Boulevard. The Silver Lake Meadow will come into view lakeside—a patch of velvety grass where you'll find couples lazing about, toddlers doing face-plants, and people flying kites. About the only thing you won't find are dogs, which are not allowed. As if to drive that point home, a sign encourages users to enjoy the meadow barefoot.

If you *did* bring Fido along on this trip, no worries, he'll get a reward in a few minutes. **Bypass the meadow by staying on Silver Lake Boulevard.** Another 1,200 steps brings you to the Silver Lake Dog Park, which includes a smaller enclosure for more timid pooches. As the hounds sniff out hindquarters, you watch for celebrities. Telltale signs are men or women with dark sunglasses and hoodies ignoring skittish Pomeranians.

PICNIC OP

Silver Lake Meadow, on Silver Lake Boulevard near Armstrong Avenue.

STEPPING BACK

Famous modern architect Richard Neutra built several residences along Silver Lake Boulevard and a nearby street called Neutra Place. To the west, another modernist, John Lautner, built his most famous home—Silver Top—on the hill across the lake. You can make out its sloping roof along the ridgeline.

From the Silver Lake Dog Park, it's just a few short steps back to your point of departure . . . and a fare-thee-well to thee.

10

GRIFFITH PARK

A RIVER RUNS THROUGH IT

One gave birth to our municipal water system; the other created the city's largest park. We honor two visionary Angelenos by splitting this route between the L.A. River and Griffith Park, pausing to admire the horses—of both the real and wooden variety.

- **TERRAIN:** Flat
- **SURFACE:** Paved and unpaved
- **FIDO FRIENDLY?:** Yes
- **PARKING:** Lot south of William Mulholland Memorial Fountain at southwest corner of Los Feliz Boulevard and Riverside Drive, or lot adjacent to Riverside Tennis Courts at 3401 Riverside Drive, Los Angeles

A case could be made that the intersection of Los Feliz Boulevard and Riverside Drive is the most historically significant in modern Los Angeles. **Begin your walk at the intersection's southwest corner,** where you'll find the William Mulholland Memorial Fountain, dedicated to the famed "father of the Los Angeles water system."

Mulholland himself lived in a nearby shack before becoming top dog of the Department of Water and Power. Since its opening in 1940, the turquoise-tiled pool with fifty-foot geysers has hosted countless weddings, quinceañeras, and photo shoots—and served as an unofficial swimming hole in hot weather.

A recent restoration has blended several new features without detracting from the fountain's Art Deco-inspired design. A

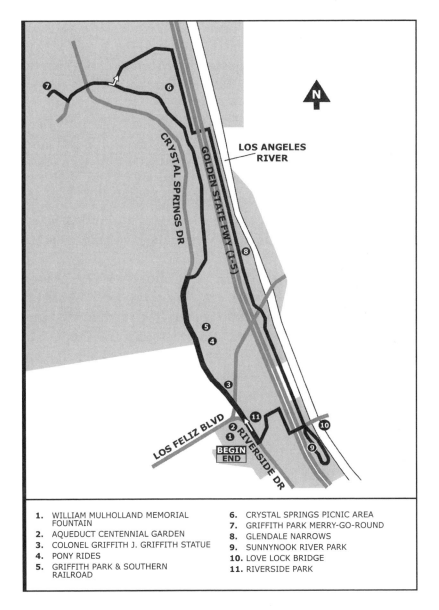

1. WILLIAM MULHOLLAND MEMORIAL FOUNTAIN
2. AQUEDUCT CENTENNIAL GARDEN
3. COLONEL GRIFFITH J. GRIFFITH STATUE
4. PONY RIDES
5. GRIFFITH PARK & SOUTHERN RAILROAD
6. CRYSTAL SPRINGS PICNIC AREA
7. GRIFFITH PARK MERRY-GO-ROUND
8. GLENDALE NARROWS
9. SUNNYNOOK RIVER PARK
10. LOVE LOCK BRIDGE
11. RIVERSIDE PARK

cross-section of pipe from Mulholland's 233-mile-long Los Angeles Aqueduct sits next to the Aqueduct Centennial Garden, while a decomposed granite walking trail ingenuously mirrors the path of the original aqueduct. If you plan on picnicking during this walk, there are even two filtered water fountains here—one for you, and another for Fido.

After ambling the fountain's grounds, cross over to the northeast corner of this intersection, which honors L.A.'s other patriarchal figure in the form of a statue. Donning a walrus mustache, Colonel Griffith Jenkins Griffith strikes a grandfatherly pose with a walking cane and a generous sweep of his hand—no doubt a gesture symbolic of his 1896 donation of thousands of acres to create Griffith Park.

Continue north on Crystal Springs Drive, staying on the right side. At 600 steps, you'll come to the parking lot for two Griffith Park institutions that have been making country bumpkins out of city kids since 1948. I rode my first horse at the Pony Rides—as did both of my children. Horse-speeds come in three varieties: "walk," "trot," and "fast jog." Next to the ponies is the Griffith Park & Southern Railroad, a miniature train ride with open-air cars that circles the southeast corner of the park. (Tip of the Day: avoid sitting directly behind the engineer unless you enjoy inhaling diesel fumes.) The one-mile track includes an old Western town with cast-off bald mannequins dressed as cowboys that will haunt your dreams.

Just north of the parking lot for the trains and ponies, **follow the dirt bridle trail that veers off the road and parallels the Golden State Freeway (I-5).** After 1,000 steps, you'll pass a massive oak tree and enter the southern portion of the Crystal Springs Picnic Area. To your right, you'll see a tunnel that goes under the freeway. Do not take that tunnel—we'll hit that on the way back. Instead,

STEPPING BACK

What you won't find on Colonel Griffith's inscription is the fact that, a few years after he gifted the land for Griffith Park, he shot his wife in the eye during a drunken rage, which many suspect led to his guilt-driven funding of the Greek Theatre and Griffith Observatory. The hotel site where the incident happened is pointed out in this book's Santa Monica walk.

bear left on the trail, which skirts the outfield of an adult baseball field and leads to a group of low-lying buildings—the park's ranger station and

> **PICNIC OP**
>
> Picnic tables are plentiful throughout Griffith Park. You can picnic either here or farther along the route.

visitors center—near the Crystal Springs parking lot entrance.

If you like, explore the visitor center. Regard its charmingly dated ceramic history of Griffith Park next to stuffed bobcats and coyotes. This is also a good spot to pick up one of those slick, colorful maps of the park.

Leaving the ranger complex, follow the sign that points to the merry-go-round across Crystal Springs Drive. Once you've crossed over, walk along the unmarked driveway for about 200 steps, then turn right on a narrow service road, proceeding another 200 paces.

The road takes you to the park's wondrous 1926 Spillman carousel where, for a few bucks, you can hop on one of its sixty-eight carved wooden horses with jeweled bridles while a vintage band organ pumps out waltzes. Walt Disney used to take his daughters on this ride, which allegedly inspired him to create Disneyland and make a carousel the centerpiece of his park, too. A bench he used sit on here is dedicated with one of his daughters' names. (Speaking of Disneyland, this merry-go-round is like an old E-ticket. It's about the fastest one you'll ever experience, so hold those reins tight and whatever you do, don't drink and ride!)

After re-establishing your equilibrium on solid ground, **retrace your steps to the unmarked driveway. Cross Crystal Springs Drive to the intersection's northeast corner and access the bridle trail on the left, heading eastward.** The trail curves to the right and hugs the wall of the Golden State Freeway. Eventually, it makes a hard left, disappearing under the freeway itself. This is the tunnel you saw earlier, a little-known wormhole that deposits you on the east

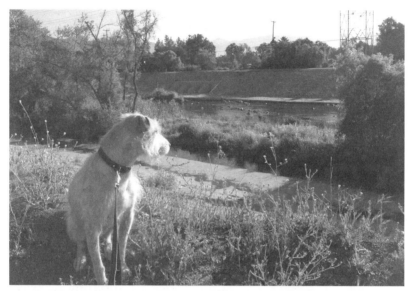

Even Porter finds the flowing waters of the Los Angeles River strangely restorative.

side of the thoroughfare.

Take the tunnel to the other side of the freeway. Trudging up a dirt ramp, you will suddenly find yourself in a whole new world along the western embankment of the Los Angeles River. Known as Glendale Narrows, this is one of those rare sections of the fifty-one-mile waterway that has a dirt bottom, its flourishing vegetation providing shelter and nourishment for birds along the Pacific Flyway. This is also, technically, still Griffith Park, which extends to the other side of the river.

Proceed south along the L.A. River bike path. Even though this is also a popular walking route, cyclists can sneak up on you, so keep an eye out! Continue past Los Feliz Boulevard—over a bridge with giant steel bicycle wheels—until you get to Sunnynook River Park. By this point, you will have walked along the river for 2,200 steps.

Loop through Sunnynook's meandering trail of interpretive signs and native plants. Circle back north

until you get to the pedestrian overpass (just north of Sunnynook River Park). One leg of the bridge heads east, where a sign points toward Atwater Village. Instead, **take the western walkway,** a fully-fenced bridge that soars over the 5 Freeway and tends to vibrate with every footstep or whooshing big rig passing inches below you. Be still, your beating heart. The bridge is not really falling . . . it only feels like it.

> **EXTRA STEPS**
>
> Doing this walk with your soul mate (and I don't mean your dog)? Bring along a lock! In a nod to the Pont des Arts bridge in Paris, the footbridge that goes over the L.A. River is now known as the Love Lock bridge. Several hundred locks are affixed to the bridge's protective fence, where only your lover has the key to your heart.

After crossing the freeway, follow the pathway as it veers sharply right to the back end of Riverside Park. Once you pass the soccer field, find the opening between the tennis courts and head toward the tennis court kiosk. (To say that this freeway bridge is hidden from view is an understatement . . . you would almost have to find it by accident if you were to enter it from this side.)

Access the walkway that takes you to the park's parking lot, where you'll find yourself directly across the street from Mulholland Fountain and the inescapable gaze of Griffith himself. Like the chastened colonel, you too have come full circle.

11

LOS FELIZ / GRIFFITH PARK

IT'S NOT ALL GREEK

This loop starts in the "figgy" foothills of Los Feliz, winds through a fern-laden wonderland, and saves the best for last on the southern slope of Mount Hollywood, where the most sought-after bodies are the planetary ones.

- **TERRAIN:** Flat and hilly
- **SURFACE:** Paved and unpaved
- **FIDO FRIENDLY?:** Yes
- **PARKING:** Street parking along Vermont Avenue, across the street from the Greek Theatre at 2700 Vermont Avenue, Los Angeles

L os Feliz is named after Mexican corporal Jose Vicente Feliz, whose rancho in the mid-nineteenth century encompassed the current boundaries of Los Feliz and Griffith Park. Rancho Los Feliz was eventually subdivided, with Griffith J. Griffith acquiring his acreage in 1882.

While these facts are indisputable, one nagging issue remains unsettled: Just what *is* the acceptable pronunciation of Los Feliz? Longtime Angelenos pronounce it with Anglicized elocution—"Las FEEL-us" (the same people who call San Pedro "San PEE-dro"). Others, sensitive to our Mexican forefathers, refer to it as "Los Feh-LEEZ." *Feliz*, of course, means "happy" in Spanish. By the time you complete this stroll through the leafy streets of Los Feliz and the endorphin-inducing trails of Griffith Park, you'll be feeling so *feliz* yourself, you really won't care what people call it.

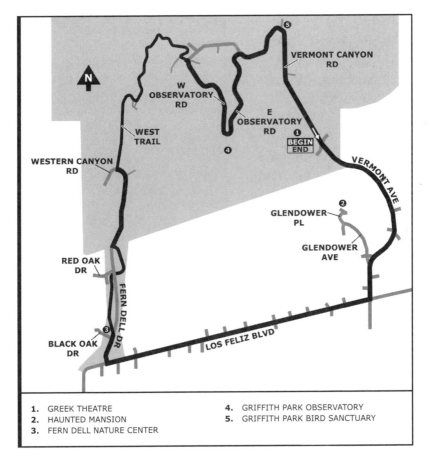

1. GREEK THEATRE
2. HAUNTED MANSION
3. FERN DELL NATURE CENTER

4. GRIFFITH PARK OBSERVATORY
5. GRIFFITH PARK BIRD SANCTUARY

Start at the front of the Greek Theatre. It's the brain-child of Colonel Griffith, who had long wanted to build an amphitheater and observatory in the park that bore his name. His trust fund ensured the completion of both in 1929 and 1935, respectively. Because it's owned by the city, you can usually roam the empty seating area during the day. A noted soprano from the 1920s—Ellen Beach Yaw—suggested that the venue be built at this site after admiring the natural acoustics of the concave canyon. Yes, I suppose that's your cue to yell "Echo!"

From the Greek, head south on Vermont Avenue into

the residential community of Los Feliz. The broad grass median is the result of a failed attempt by Colonel Griffith to convince the Pacific Electric Company to extend a trolley into his park. At the 1,000-step mark, you'll start to feel very small. Are you shrinking? No, it's just your surroundings—massive 100-year-old Moreton Bay fig trees that buckle the sidewalk and look ripped straight out of *Jack and the Beanstalk*. Cumulatively, the trees are a Historic-Cultural Monument.

EXTRA STEPS

Wanna see a haunted house? As you head down Vermont, make a right on Glendower Avenue, then another right at Glendower Place. The mansion at 2475 was the site of a grisly murder-suicide in 1959. Though no one has occupied it since then—unopened Christmas presents and 1950s board games are still visible through the front window—ghosts have reportedly taken up residence. If these spiritual inhabitants ever feel motivated to sell, the 5,000 square foot estate should fetch them upwards of $3.5 million.

Not to be outdone, the deodar cedars along Los Feliz Boulevard also enjoy Historic-Cultural status. They form a cool canopy as you **head west on Los Feliz along its northern greenbelt,** and were planted by the Los Feliz Women's Club around the same time as the fig trees.

After 2,000 steps on Los Feliz, you'll reach Fern Dell Drive. On your right, you'll see a statue of a bear donated by L.A.'s sister city—Berlin, Germany. There, the bear is a 700-year-old symbol of strength and resiliency. Here, he's a convenient plaything for random acts of dress-up. Over the years, mischief-makers have decked him out in various bewildering ensembles, including Santa Claus. In my humble opinion, the pink tutu suited him best.

Cross over to the west side of Fern Dell, where you'll find another gifted statue, this one by the Los Angeles-Norwegian community. Say hello to Leif Erikson, the famed Viking adventurer. The monument makes a point of asserting that he landed in America 492 years before Christopher Columbus. I don't know about you, but I detect a little sour grapes from the Norwegians.

Ditching Herr Erikson, **proceed one block north on Fern Dell, re-entering Griffith Park.** Look for the wooden sign marking the entrance to the Fern Dell (also written as "Ferndell") Nature Center, where Black Oak Drive meets Fern Dell Drive. A marker in the ground designates the area as a sacred spot for the Tongva/Gabrielino Indians, who were drawn to its year-round spring.

Enter through the gates of the Nature Center. A crooked dirt pathway will take you through a dense forest dominated by giant ferns and redwoods. Construction began on Fern Dell in 1914, but landscaping continued over the next two decades, with benches, bridges, and terraced pools added by the Civilian Conservation Corps. By the 1930s, Fern Dell emerged as a must-see L.A. destination, its image burnished on post-cards ("50 Species of Ferns!"). These days, signs of deferred maintenance are everywhere, but its sense of wonder remains, and it's still the coolest spot in Griffith Park on a hot summer's day. Find yourself a nice stony nook and relax alongside a gurgling waterfall, keeping an eye out for frogs.

> **PICNIC OP**
>
> Fern Dell Nature Center, west-adjacent to Fern Dell Drive.

Continue through Fern Dell as it goes under Fern Dell Drive and ends on the east side of the street. Continue along the elevated post-and-beam nature path that parallels Fern Dell Drive. If you didn't pack a picnic—heck, even if you did—you must visit the Trails Café, one block north of Red Oak Drive on the west side of Fern Dell Drive (which turns into Western Canyon Road). Housed in an old wooden park building that was deeded to termites, it's taken on new life as a haven for hungry hikers. Park yourself on a bale of hay in their woodsy outdoor seating area and enjoy the simple pleasure of an avocado-with-sprouts sandwich, or a piece of freshly baked pie and lemonade.

From Trails Café, head up Western Canyon Road for about 400 steps, at which point the street makes a hairpin turn. At the top of the hairpin is a dirt fire trail known as West Trail that's heavily used by hikers. **Access West Trail,** which heads into a chaparral-filled canyon. **Five hundred steps up, follow the trail as it does its own hairpin turn, to the right. Turn left at the T-intersection, heading north, then hike another 1,000 steps up the hillside. Bear left near the top of the trail to access W. Observatory Road,** which takes cars up to the Griffith Park Observatory. **Hang a right onto that street's sidewalk.**

In about 600 steps, the inviting front lawn of the Griffith Park Observatory will spread out before you. The Observatory's copper dome has become a signature icon of Los Angeles, much like the Hollywood Sign, which can be seen off to the right. At the center of the lawn is another magnificent sculpture built under the auspices of the WPA—the Astronomers Monument, which celebrates six of the world's greatest astronomers.

Unlike most observatories, the Griffith Observatory was built more for the public than for astronomers. The education begins on the sidewalk leading up to the entrance. It depicts the orbits of the planets in our solar system relative to one another, starting with Pluto on the outer edge. Despite being kicked out of the planetary club in 2006 by the International Astronomical Union, Hollywood loves a good underdog story, so Pluto is still recognized by the Observatory!

The stars in the sky, of course, aren't the only ones visible from up here. **Cross over to the western sidewalk** and fist-bump the bust of one James Dean. Several key scenes from 1955's *Rebel Without a Cause* were shot at the Griffith Observatory. **Continue past Dean's bust and circle the Observatory via its outdoor viewing areas.** Gazing out at the basin from your Art Deco aerie as a gentle breeze softens the sun's rays, you find yourself experiencing what I like to call "an L.A. moment." The view is simply breathtak-

STEPPING BACK

During World War II, the Observatory's planetarium was co-opted by the military. They used it to help teach naval aviators how to navigate by the stars.

ing, its expansiveness hinting toward the city's endless possibilities, instilling optimism in even the most hardened critic.

There is plenty more inspiration to find inside the Observatory, but given its scope, that's a visit for another day. **Find your way back to the front of the Observatory. Just past its front lawn, access E. Observatory Road, the roadway to the right that goes downhill. At the 600-step mark, turn right onto Vermont Canyon Road.** As you do, glance over your shoulder at the 1927-built tunnel. It was featured in the chase scene from *Who Framed Roger Rabbit!*

After 300 steps, Vermont Canyon makes a sharp right turn. On the left side of the street, you'll see a sign for the Griffith Park Bird Sanctuary, opened in 1922 by the Audubon Society (which recruited Boy Scouts to build its culvert and bridges). Throughout the years, though, it's never lived up to its billing; you'll find more birds hanging out in your backyard. Still, anything from the 1920s "back to nature" conservation movement—a carry-over from Theodore Roosevelt's era—is ultimately worth hanging onto.

From the Bird Sanctuary, it's another 300 steps back to the Greek Theatre. The amphitheater's marquee is advertising the Doobie Brothers, and roadies are unloading gear from a luxury bus. You've already had your high—best to clear out before the invasion of aging hippies have theirs.

12

LOS ANGELES RIVER

RAPIDS TRANSIT DISTRICT

There was a time when no one in L.A. would sing "Take Me to the River," but the city has changed its tune regarding the eponymous waterway. This up-and-back showcases the river's wild side, with stops along five riverside parklets.

- **TERRAIN:** Flat
- **SURFACE:** Mostly paved
- **FIDO FRIENDLY?:** Yes
- **PARKING:** Street parking near Oso Park at the intersection of Oros Street and Blake Avenue, Los Angeles

Over the course of the twentieth century, the Los Angeles River went from a lifeline to a punchline. Once an important water source for early inhabitants, the river lost its purpose after William Mulholland turned on the spigot for the Los Angeles Aqueduct in 1913. By the second half of the century it was relegated to cameos in movies like *Grease* and *Volcano*. But thanks to the efforts of organizations like Friends of the L.A. River, the river is relevant again. This portion east of the Golden State Freeway (I-5) provides a preview of its full recreational potential.

From its junction with Oros Street, head south on Blake Avenue, accessing the short walking trail separating Blake from Riverside Drive. It's part of Oso Park, certainly one of the smallest parks in the entire Santa Monica Mountains Conservancy. In addition to native trees, the

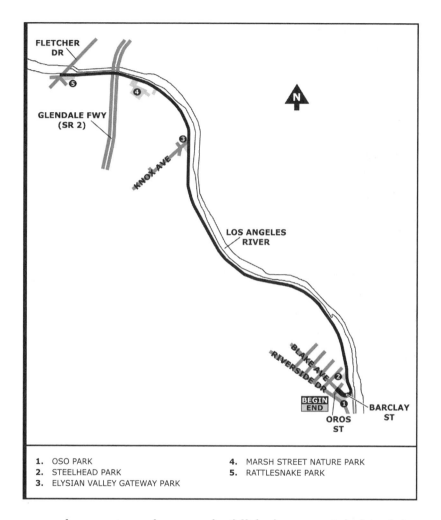

1. OSO PARK
2. STEELHEAD PARK
3. ELYSIAN VALLEY GATEWAY PARK
4. MARSH STREET NATURE PARK
5. RATTLESNAKE PARK

grounds contain sculptures of wildlife that once inhabited the river, offering a nice prelude to this walk.

Follow Blake as it bends toward the river (technically becoming Barclay Street). At the end of Barclay, go through the entrance to the Los Angeles River Greenway Trail. A green directional sign points to three destinations to the left. One of them is Fletcher Drive at 2.5 miles. Since 5,000 steps equals 2.5 miles, Fletcher will be your turnaround point. Though you may be tempted to turn right, know that the trail dead-ends in a few hundred yards once it reaches the Figueroa Street Bridge (there are plans to extend the pathway through downtown).

Turning left, journey along the river's western embankment. As always with shared bike/walk paths, look out for cyclists, who zip along at pretty decent clips. After a mere 400 feet—where Oros Street dead-ends at the river—you'll come to Steelhead Park. The park's rust-colored gate is adorned with leaping steelhead trout, once plentiful in L.A.'s natural waterways. River advocates hope the fish will eventually find their way back up the river from the ocean, rejoining other species that already call it home.

Access Steelhead Park's short walkway. Note the sign that reads "Los Angeles River Recreational Zone." Steelhead Park is the southernmost point of the navigational stretch that starts at Fletcher. On summer weekends, the river is open to any Angeleno wanting to steer a boat, kayak, or canoe down the channel. Bring your own water transport or rent one through an authorized company.

Continue north up the pathway. Pass a mural featuring a frog dressed in an "I ♥ the L.A. River" T-shirt who happily discards a car tire during one of the river's volunteer cleanups. This portion of the waterway is part of a six-mile section with a natural bottom. Long-term goals are to rip out the concrete basin in much of the fifty-one-mile river, which was paved over by the Army Corps of Engineers after the devastating floods of 1938. The advantages of a natural river are plain to see. Islands of willows, cottonwoods, and alders create rapids for boaters, while large birds swoop in to snatch a carp or largemouth bass.

Three thousand steps from Steelhead Park is Elysian Valley Gateway Park, with plenty of trees and grass. After another 600 steps, you'll come to Marsh Street Nature Park, which includes L.A. River-based animal sculptures for kids to climb.

Continue north under the Glendale Freeway (SR 2)

to the fifth and final greenbelt of the Elysian Valley zone—Rattlesnake Park, named after a bed of rattlesnakes

PICNIC OP

Elysian Valley Gateway Park, adjacent to the river at the terminus of Knox Avenue.

found there when the park was constructed. Located just south of the historic Fletcher Drive Bridge, it serves as the northernmost entry point for boaters wishing to access the river at Rattlesnake Rapids. Note the snake motifs in the stonework and rock wall. The park also includes an illustrated history of Juan Bautista de Anza's 1775 expedition to Paime Pahite ("Western River" in Tongva), which is accompanied by a stone marker designating the river a National Historic Trail.

You've now reached the halfway point—time to turn around. They say de Anza walked more than 1,000 miles from Mexico to get to this river. That's roughly 2,000,000 steps. Suddenly, walking another 5,000 back to your car doesn't feel so ominous . . .

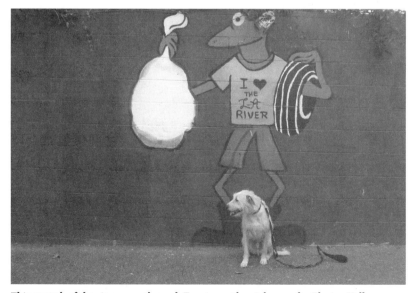

This stretch of the river runs through Frogtown, the nickname for Elysian Valley.

13

EAGLE ROCK

BEYOND THE BOULDER

Eagle Rock: its name somehow sounds both whimsical and dignified, setting the perfect tone for a jaunt among fairy-tale houses and Historic-Cultural Monuments. And, oh yeah, the most famous rock this side of Plymouth.

- ■ **TERRAIN:** Flat with slight inclines
- ■ **SURFACE:** Mostly paved
- ■ **FIDO FRIENDLY?:** Yes
- ■ **PARKING:** Street parking near Richard Alatorre Park at 7608 Scholl Canyon Road, Eagle Rock

It's the only rock in Los Angeles to have achieved Historic-Cultural status, giving hope to billions of aspirational boulders everywhere. It is, of course, Eagle Rock.

The best place to view Eagle Rock is at this walk's origin—Richard Alatorre Park at 7608 Scholl Canyon Road, which is basically a continuation of Figueroa Street just north of the Ventura Freeway (SR 134). The park itself is no great shakes, but you've come for the view.

A few yards east is the massive bald crag in the flesh. When the sun hits just right, an indentation on the rock casts

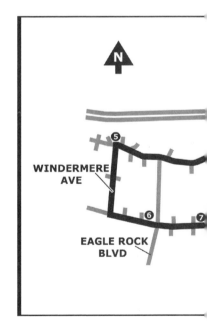

a shadow that looks like an eagle taking flight, giving it—and the community—its name.

With the rock behind us, it's time to invade the neighborhood. From the park, **head south on Scholl Canyon Road under the freeway overpass, then west on Eagle Vista Drive.** On your left is one of the largest public parks in L.A.—the Eagle Rock Recreation Center, tucked between the freeway and the surrounding streets. As Eagle Vista bends around the park, notice the boxy gymnasium that looks like a giant children's toy. It was designed by architect Richard Neutra in 1953 and has since been awarded landmark status. **Take a quick excursion through the park, using a short, shady nature trail that loops behind the gym. Return to**

1. RICHARD ALATORRE PARK
2. EAGLE ROCK
3. EAGLE ROCK RECREATION CENTER
4. MILO BEKINS CHATEAU
5. MATT DAMON AND BEN AFFLECK RESIDENCE (FORMER LOCATION)
6. EAGLE ROCK LIBRARY (FORMER LOCATION)
7. EAGLE ROCK CITY HALL (FORMER LOCATION)
8. WOMEN'S TWENTIETH CENTURY CLUB OF EAGLE ROCK
9. HAPPY CAMP

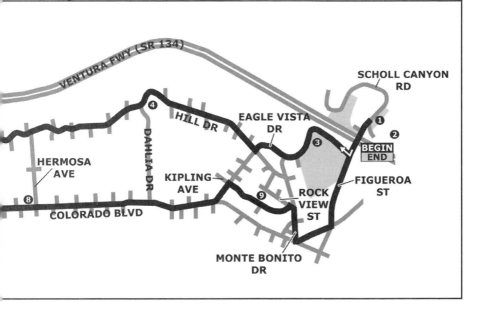

Eagle Vista and follow it down to Hill Drive.
  Turn right on Hill, heading west. The

> **PICNIC OP**
> Eagle Rock Recreation Center, 1100 Eagle Vista Drive.

street parallels Colorado Boulevard and goes through a stately residential section. Things really get interesting around the 2,500-step mark, where Hill intersects Dahlia Drive. On the southeast corner is an imposing manor that lords over the neighborhood from its hilly roost. Known as the Chateau, it was built in 1925 for Milo Bekins of Bekins Storage fame. It once hosted a presidential address by Ronald Reagan. But the grand dame looks tired, and its terraced grounds are so jungly, you half-expect howler monkeys to leap out, lending a certain *Grey Gardens* vibe to the whole thing.

Stick to the north sidewalk as you continue west on Hill. Towering palms begin to line the street. Houses are marked by small stone walls fronting rambling yards with mature trees supporting treehouses, rope swings, and hammocks. The styles are quintessential L.A.—a mix of Craftsman, Neoclassical, and mid-century modern. Hard to believe that the 134 Freeway is less than 1,000 feet to your right. But thanks to the fact that it's uphill from here, you barely notice its noise.

At 2327 Hill—the walk's halfway point—is a medieval-inspired chateau with crooked arches and white stucco walls with dark wood trim. The fairy-tale motifs seem appropriate, since its former tenants were a couple of young men with charmed lives. For it is here that roommates Matt Damon and Ben Affleck wrote the screenplay for their Oscar-winning movie *Good Will Hunting* while Affleck was attending Occidental College. A sign identifies the structure as a Historic-Cultural Landmark. Nothing against the former occupants, but even their star status is not enough to warrant this special designation. The 1923 house honors the collaborative vision of its original owner, Albert Braasch, and his architect, J. L. Egasse.

Directly across the street from this house is Windermere

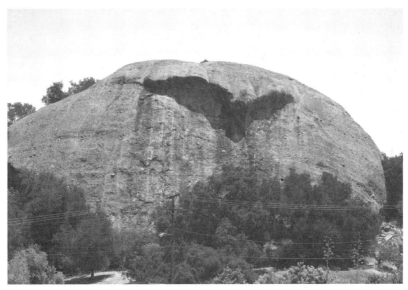

The "eagle" of Eagle Rock only appears when the sun hits it just right.

Avenue. **Proceed two blocks down Windemere until you get to Colorado. Make a left on Colorado, sticking to the north sidewalk.** As you buzz along Eagle Rock's main thoroughfare, you'll pass a number of yummy eateries east of Eagle Rock Boulevard. The Oinkster—outfitted in the A-framed shell of an old Der Wienerschnitzel—is known for its slow-cooked pastrami. You will also come across a number of other Historic-Cultural Monuments, including the original Eagle Rock Library (2225 Colorado) and Eagle Rock City Hall (2035 Colorado), both built in the 1920s in the Mission Revival style.

Two blocks past City Hall, on the corner of Colorado and Hermosa Avenue, is perhaps the most significant building in Eagle Rock. The Women's Twentieth Century Club of Eagle Rock meets in a handsome Craftsman clubhouse that looks much the same as it did when it opened its doors over 100 years ago. Like a lot of women's clubs in the early twentieth century, the ladies helped push for women's suffrage and equality. **Continue another 1,400 steps along Colorado, then**

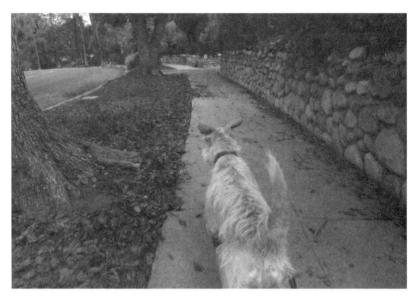

Porter on "squirrel alert" as he romps along Hill Drive.

turn left on Eagle Vista Drive, re-entering the residential region. One block up, turn right on Kipling Avenue. At 1203 is a colorful cottage known as "Happy Camp" that looks like something out of *Hansel and Gretel*. It was built by movie set designer Howard Edwards in the early 1920s, an era that saw the construction of other playful structures like the Egasse-Braasch house, and two built by a fellow set designer, Harry Oliver: the Witch's House in Beverly Hills, and the Tam O'Shanter restaurant in Los Feliz.

Continue on Kipling until it hits Rock View

STEPPING BACK

Heading south on Monte Bonito and north on Figueroa, you will pass under a split overpass serving cars that enter and exit the 134 Freeway. This bridge is a vestige of the old Colorado Freeway. It was replaced by the Ventura Freeway in 1971, but segments of the former freeway remain, including its western terminus, where Colorado Boulevard turns into a mini-freeway between San Fernando Road and the Golden State Freeway (I-5) in Glendale.

Street. Make a right, then another quick right onto Monte Bonito Drive, which takes you back to Colorado. Hang a left on Colorado. After one block, go left on Figueroa until you pass under the freeway. Relocate the Richard Alatorre Park on your right. If you're lucky, the eagle will still be soaring above you just a few yards away.

Overleaf: Residents of MacArthur Park Lake in Westlake.

HOLLYWOOD
AND MID-CITY

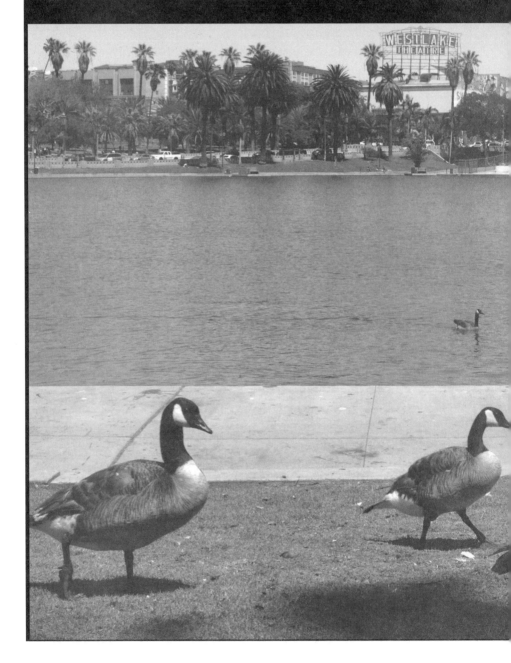

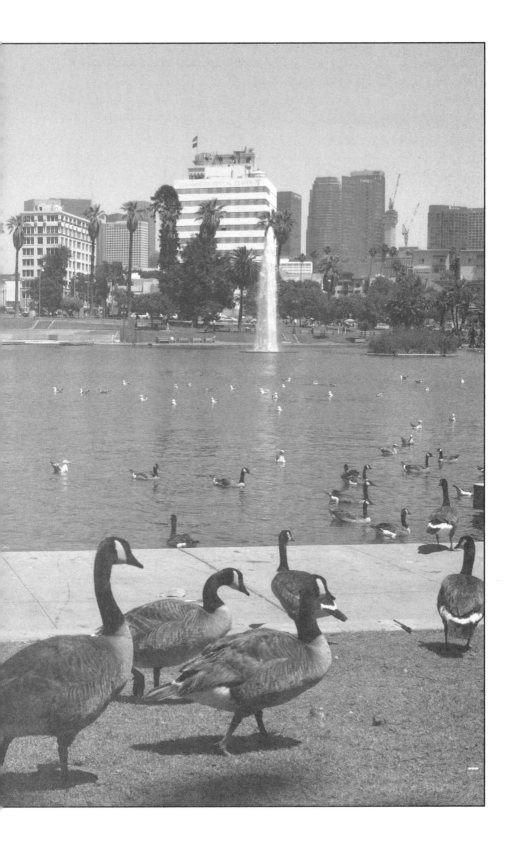

14

HOLLYWOOD

HIDING IN PLAIN SIGHT

*Ever had the feeling you were being watched? You will
on this "anti-tourist" walk along Hollywood Boulevard
. . . but it's not as creepy as you think. P.S. Don't forget
to bring along binoculars.*

- **TERRAIN:** Flat
- **SURFACE:** Paved
- **FIDO FRIENDLY?:** Yes
- **PARKING:** Street parking on side streets, near the
  intersection of Hollywood Boulevard and Western
  Avenue

I n the 1920s, Hollywood Boulevard was the West Coast's
answer to New York's Great White Way. Architects
bathed movie theaters, nightclubs, and office buildings

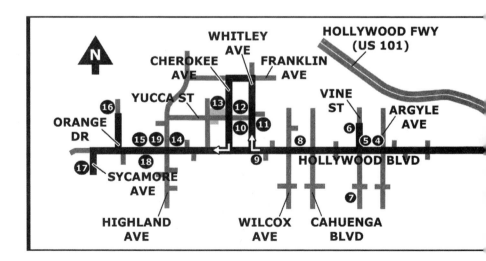

in a quixotic sheen of influences, creating monuments of opulence that appealed to Hollywood's outsized sense of self. Architectural purists may have fainted at this clash of styles, but in a frontier town like L.A., they found a place where Old World rules happily came to die.

Central to many of these historic edifices are perhaps the most intricate, yet overlooked, flourishes of architecture in Los Angeles: sculpted faces—human, beast, and otherworldly—embedded in their facades. There are literally hundreds of them on the two-mile stretch of Hollywood Boulevard between Western and La Brea Avenues. Some are playfully defiant. Others cast a stony gaze upon passersby in silent yearning. A wizened few seem resigned to their purgatory, eyes glazed over with indifference. All of them are remnants of a more glamorous era, eternally ready for their close-up. And while this walk covers the best of them, keep an eye out for others not covered here.

Start at the southwest corner of Western and Hollywood, the site of the historic Mayer Building, designed by S. Charles Lee and built by Louis B. Mayer. In my twenties, when Hollywood Billiards was a tenant, I whiled away nights playing

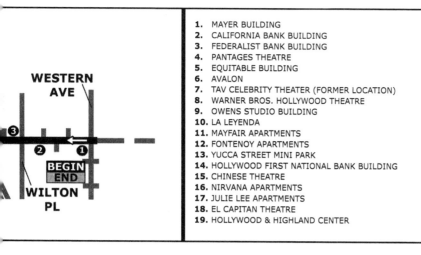

WESTERN
AVE

BEGIN
END
WILTON
PL

1. MAYER BUILDING
2. CALIFORNIA BANK BUILDING
3. FEDERALIST BANK BUILDING
4. PANTAGES THEATRE
5. EQUITABLE BUILDING
6. AVALON
7. TAV CELEBRITY THEATER (FORMER LOCATION)
8. WARNER BROS. HOLLYWOOD THEATRE
9. OWENS STUDIO BUILDING
10. LA LEYENDA
11. MAYFAIR APARTMENTS
12. FONTENOY APARTMENTS
13. YUCCA STREET MINI PARK
14. HOLLYWOOD FIRST NATIONAL BANK BUILDING
15. CHINESE THEATRE
16. NIRVANA APARTMENTS
17. JULIE LEE APARTMENTS
18. EL CAPITAN THEATRE
19. HOLLYWOOD & HIGHLAND CENTER

pool in its dingy basement, never realizing that the 1928 landmark had once hosted the offices of Cecil B. DeMille and Central Casting—a company so large that we regularly invoke its name when we talk about a clichéd movie character "straight out of Central Casting." But it was another tenant that wielded more influence than anyone on

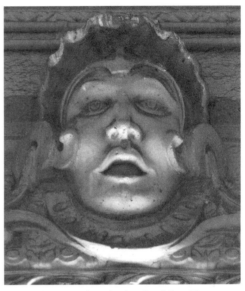

Spooky thespians line the façade of the old Warner Bros. Theatre at Hollywood and Wilcox.

motion pictures. The Hays Office governed cinematic morality for close to forty years before the MPAA rating system took over in 1968. The building's plaster-finished fire escapes cleverly comment on the thorny issue of censorship, with dozens of intertwined nude figures engaged in a tug-of-war in front of camera crews. On the underside of the escapes, an equally naked Mercury delivers a film canister. Can you imagine a structure being approved today with this much public nudity?

As you **continue west on Hollywood Boulevard,** walk along the northern sidewalk to get a better view of the deific portraits along the building's cornice. Meanwhile, hovering above the main entryway is . . . who is that? Moses? Poseidon? Old Man Winter? As with many of the buildings you're about to see, it really doesn't matter. Playfulness is the name of the game here; whimsy and creative boldness, the only rules.

Several blocks west, at 5620 Hollywood, is an Art Deco tower from 1929. Originally built for the California Bank, it stood in as a movie theater in *L.A. Confidential.* A very regal eagle sits prominently above the door. Eagles were important symbols of strength for banks, especially those built after the stock market crash of 1929.

One block west, on the northwest corner of Hollywood and Wilton Place, an escrow company occupies the site of the old Federalist Bank Building from 1930. Perched above the 5701 address is a sculpture of an eagle, proudly flexing its wings. Speaking of which, look for the winged lions in the frieze that bends around the corner. They're a common motif in many structures along this corridor.

Proceed 1,600 steps to Hollywood and Argyle Avenue. At 6233 Hollywood is the Pantages Theatre, the well-known Art Deco citadel from 1930. The converted movie house regularly showcases the hottest Broadway plays. If you can't get into the lobby—gleaming metallic shades flanked by gilded statues and a sweeping staircase—you can at least admire the golden pharaohs gazing down from the cornice.

Less appreciated is the 1929 high-rise just west of the Pantages, on the northeast corner of Hollywood and Vine Street. The Equitable Building has several random faces hiding out in its otherwise Classical walls. Look for the pissed-off bearded fellow who bears a striking resemblance to Gollum from *The Lord of the Rings*. Turn the corner onto Vine, and you'll find fifteen corbel figures buttressing a fifth floor balcony.

Continue half a block north on Vine, then take the crosswalk to the Avalon club at 1735 Vine. How many of us have caught a show here at night and never noticed the myriad figures flanking its plastered entrance? It's only in the revealing light of day that we realize just how nightmarish they really are—goat-men

STEPPING BACK

Howard Hughes bought the Pantages in 1949 as part of his RKO movie theater chain. The notoriously reclusive billionaire certainly hasn't been shy in the afterlife. Many employees swear that his ghost haunts his old offices on the second floor of the building.

and sphinxes mingling with buxom she-dragons and maniacal hucksters who look like the wizard from the land of Oz.

Head back to Hollywood Boulevard and turn right.
Just past Cahuenga Boulevard (at 6423 Hollywood) is the old Warner Bros. Hollywood Theatre. Warners' *The Jazz Singer* was the first feature-length "talkie" in 1927, and this theater—christened a year later—was the first on the West Coast to be wired for sound. Architect G. Albert Lansburgh lined its exterior with no less than seventy-five faces representing the dramatic arts, a motley menagerie of plutocrats, cherubs, and demonic cats. My favorite is a dragon-serpent set in a swirl of plaster under the archway leading to the building's lobby. Even the theater's exit doors along Wilcox are

> **EXTRA STEPS**
>
> ABC's former West Coast headquarters, which later became the TAV Celebrity Theater—home to *The Merv Griffin Show*—lies at 1533 Vine, a block and a half south of Hollywood Boulevard. A fire gutted the building in the 1990s, but the façade was preserved in the mixed-use complex that's there now. Look for the etchings of actors and movie crews carved into the plaster walls supporting the residential units above the courtyard.

special, lorded over by actors donning masks. You won't find touches like this at your local cineplex.

Continue a block and a half past Wilcox, staying on the north side of Hollywood—the optimal side to view the old Owens Studio Building at 6554, where a Churrigueresque tableau sits above a series of Moorish arches. Buried in its swirling ornamentation are dozens of figures—an exact count depends on your perceptiveness—resulting in a "Where's Waldo?" orgy of grotesque masks, deities, elephants, and ogres. This is definitely a good time to bust out your binoculars. Even the façade's sprouting plants have tiny, embryonic figurines crawling within them—nearly impossible to see with the naked eye.

Portraits don't only live on Hollywood Boulevard's commercial buildings. To continue the treasure hunt, **venture right on Whitley Avenue.**

> **PICNIC OP**
> Yucca Street Mini Park, on the northwest corner of Cherokee Avenue and Yucca Street.

Look for visages peeking out from several historic apartment towers, including the La Leyenda at 1737 (jesters, beasts, and cherubs), the Mayfair at 1760 (winged lions, mermaids, and Neptune), and the Fontenoy at 1811 (a lonely maiden). **At Franklin Avenue, turn left. After one block, turn left again on Cherokee Avenue,** which takes you back to Hollywood Boulevard.

Turn right on Hollywood Boulevard. After 500 steps, you'll reach the northeast corner of Hollywood and Highland, where the Hollywood First National Bank Building languishes in the shadow of the monstrous mall across the street. Designed by the same firm that built the Chinese and Egyptian Theatres, it was briefly the tallest high-rise in L.A. when it opened in 1927. Some of its best sculptures are above the sixth floor, including a pious Saint Thomas Aquinas and various Gothic gargoyles (the eastern patio of the Hollywood & Highland Center affords a bird's-eye view). Closer to street level are beautiful bas-reliefs of Columbus and Copernicus representing various human achievements. And for good measure, the two-headed Roman god Janus makes a cameo.

Since this walk is a decidedly "anti-tourist" one, it would be best to power past the Chinese Theatre, lest you want to be accosted by Spider-Man and other superheroes looking for photo ops. However, **turn the corner from the Chinese Theatre** to find, fittingly, an Oriental Revival apartment complex at 1775 Orange Drive. Built in 1925, the Nirvana is graced with Chinese figures and a hand-carved dragon above the front entrance.

From there, **head back to Hollywood, walk one block to the right, and then turn left to reach another apart-**

ment building at 1665 Sycamore. The Julie Lee was built one year after the Nirvana, but her guardians have not aged nearly as well. In the upper corners, facing Sycamore, are fetching young lasses bearing bowls of fruit above their heads. Unfortunately, the masonry on one of the corners has completely stripped away, exposing the brick. The other corner statuette is rapidly crumbling, and may even be gone by the time you read this.

Like the Julie Lee, the El Capitan Theatre's figurines were also once on the verge of extinction. To get there, **head back to Hollywood Boulevard and go one block east.** The Spanish Baroque cinema has an intricate Churrigueresque façade, which requires constant upkeep due to its minute detail. By the late 1980s, the structure was as seedy as Hollywood at the time, and was dealt a further blow when it was briefly red-tagged after the 1994 Northridge Quake. Fortunately, the Disney company carefully restored it to its former glory and then some. The colored faces in its vestibule explode in funhouse revelry that stops just short of tacky. Its walls are tricked out with sepia-toned royalty types and cherubs grabbing the tails

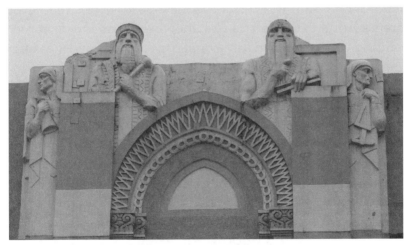

True to its origins, the Central Casting building at Hollywood and Western is festooned with interesting characters.

of winged tigers within an iron colonnade. Even the wooden columns under the marquee are, upon closer inspection, actually totems hiding even more faces. Like those on the First National Building, the portraits at the top of the theater are best appreciated from the Hollywood & Highland Center—in this case, the southern patio.

It's 3,800 steps back to your point of origin at Hollywood and Western. As you watch the tourists fix their gazes at the 2,400 stars along the Hollywood Walk of Fame, your field of vision has been forever changed. For you now know that the real treasures come from looking up.

15

HOLLYWOOD HEIGHTS / WHITLEY HEIGHTS

REACHING OLD HEIGHTS

Old Hollywood may have faded away, but its legacy shines on in Hollywood Heights and Whitley Heights. This sightseeing tour includes an old silent-movie studio, a fairy-tale castle, a tower fit for a gumshoe, and Oscar's little-known female cousin.

- **TERRAIN:** Flat and hilly with stairs
- **SURFACE:** Mostly paved
- **FIDO FRIENDLY?:** Yes
- **PARKING:** Lot for Hollywood & Highland Center, at 6801 Hollywood Boulevard, Hollywood

Long before Hollywood's glitterati started settling in Westside enclaves like Bel-Air, Pacific Palisades, and Malibu, Hollywood had its own hillside hideaways. Hollywood Heights and Whitley Heights were mere minutes from the studios and close enough for stars like Rudolph Valentino to stumble home from speakeasies along Hollywood Boulevard.

The first thing you'll want to do is escape the tourist frenzy that is Hollywood & Highland as fast as you can. **From the junction of Highland Avenue and Franklin Place, head west on Franklin Avenue.** At 7001 is a chateau-style mansion that houses the Magic Castle, a private club where magicians put on nightly shows. If you don't belong to the Academy of Magical Arts, fear not. Springing for a room at the adjacent Magic Castle Hotel comes with admission for one night at the Magic Castle, where you can roam from room

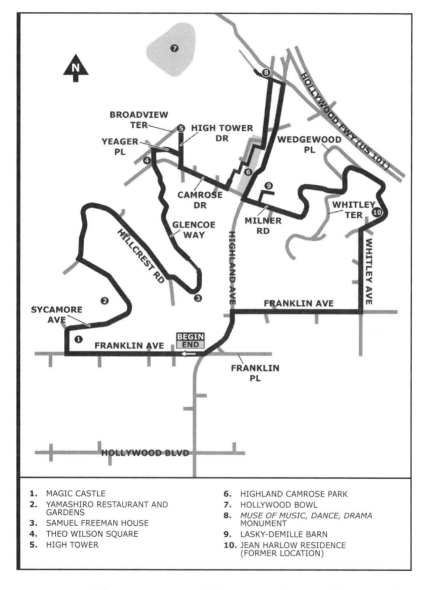

1. MAGIC CASTLE
2. YAMASHIRO RESTAURANT AND GARDENS
3. SAMUEL FREEMAN HOUSE
4. THEO WILSON SQUARE
5. HIGH TOWER
6. HIGHLAND CAMROSE PARK
7. HOLLYWOOD BOWL
8. *MUSE OF MUSIC, DANCE, DRAMA* MONUMENT
9. LASKY-DEMILLE BARN
10. JEAN HARLOW RESIDENCE (FORMER LOCATION)

to room and have your mind blown by the world's best illusionists. This is one of those L.A. bucket list items you'll be really glad you checked off.

Just past the Magic Castle Hotel is a sign for Yamashiro Restaurant pointing up Sycamore Avenue. **Make a right on**

Sycamore, then another quick right as the street be-comes one-way. Follow Sycamore as it loops around Ya-mashiro Restaurant and Gardens. Like the Magic Castle, this is another century-old venue worth visiting at night (for years it was my go-to spot to bring dates, who were always more impressed by the views than by my company). Built by hundreds of craftsmen from the Orient, the complex was pat-terned after a palace in Kyoto, Japan. Its terraced garden in-cludes a 600-year-old pagoda.

Staying on Sycamore, continue past the Yamashi-ro driveway, entering the residential region of Hollywood Heights. After a sharp right, Sycamore turns into Hillcrest Road. **Turn left at Glencoe Way,** which climbs a hill. Keep an eye out for the Samuel Freeman House at 1962 Glencoe. The landmark 1924 home was designed by Frank Lloyd Wright and features his signature textile blocks.

A couple hundred feet past the Wright house, Glencoe dead-ends—for cars, at least. **Just past the garage at address 1983, access the fifteen steps that look like they lead to a private residence.** Trust me, these are public stairs! They lead to a shaded, little-known passageway between several houses that lets out on the *other* side of Glencoe Way, which is accessible to vehicular traffic. You are now a streetwalker again. Be sure to appreciate the panoramic views of the Holly-wood Hills to your right.

Walk down Glen-coe until it intersects Camrose Drive. A city sign designates this in-tersection as Theo Wil-son Square, named af-ter a longtime resident who helped preserve the integrity of Hollywood Heights. **Continue one**

> **EXTRA STEPS**
>
> To the left of Yeager Place is a sign marking Broadview Terrace, which leads to a community called Alta Loma that is only accessible via this pedestrian walkway (or the High Tower elevator; see below). Though there are multiple exit points, I would suggest doubling back so as not to get lost. It will add about 1,000 steps.

more block to Yeager Place, and witness what Theo was fighting for. The whole area feels like a small Mediterranean village.

Make a right on Yeager Place, then turn left on High Tower Drive and walk to the end of the street. The commanding presence in front of you is High Tower—a private, five-story elevator that leads to the homes of Alta Loma. The campanile-style structure has appeared in several movies since its construction in the early 1920s, most notably in Robert Altman's *The Long Goodbye*, in which Elliott Gould's Philip Marlowe has to fend off topless girls who just want to get stoned. It was 1973, after all.

Double back on High Tower Drive to Camrose. Follow Camrose downhill. Just before you get to Highland, find the entrance to Highland Camrose Park on your left, an in-the-know micropark for pre-Hollywood Bowl concert pic-

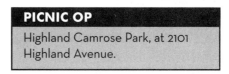

PICNIC OP

Highland Camrose Park, at 2101 Highland Avenue.

nickers (and regular ones!) drawn by its numerous tables and trellises. A nice surprise in this park is its Bungalow Village. Part of the National Register of Historic Places, the Craftsmans host the offices of the L.A. Philharmonic Orchestra and the Sheriff's Department. Do you think deputies ever tell them to keep the music down?

Exit the park at its northern gate and go left on Highland. Just before the Hollywood Bowl sign, turn left on a walkway that leads to the Bowl—the largest natural amphitheater in the nation. Legend has it that when a wooden fence was built along this walkway, the posts took root and grew into pepper trees, earning it the name Peppertree Lane (and reinforcing Hollywood as a place that thrives on mythmaking). To the left of the remaining pepper trees is the Hollywood Bowl Museum, which documents decades' worth of performances through audio, video, and print. It's worth a visit for the admission price alone—free! Check out the Beatles exhibit on the second floor.

As for the Bowl itself, seeing a show here is always a transformative experience. Although that's more of a nighttime activity, the county-run venue does famously open its doors on certain summer days, allowing Angelenos to eavesdrop on the Philharmonic conducting its rehearsals.

As you depart the Bowl, be sure to honor the *Muse of Music, Dance, Drama* monument, located to the left of the Hollywood Bowl sign near the exit. Built in 1940, it was designed by sculptor George Stanley, the same guy who created the Oscar statuette.

In front of the monument, there's a pedestrian walkway that leads underground. **Take this tunnel to the east side of Highland and head south to Milner Road.**

On the northeast corner of Milner and Highland is a parking lot. **Step onto the lot and head over to the clapboard house about 100 yards**

> **SIDE-STEP**
>
> Sometimes the pedestrian tunnel is locked during non-concert hours. If that's the case, simply return to Camrose Drive via Highland. Cross Highland at street-level, going east, to get to Milner Road.

in the distance. Built in 1895, the Lasky-Demille Barn was one of Hollywood's first studios. The building's current tenant is the preservation society Hollywood Heritage, which curates an excellent on-site museum that features silent-movie memorabilia.

From the barn, start your climb up Milner into Whitley Heights—not just the first celebrity-centric hood in L.A. but, really, the first to embrace our city's Mediterranean climate and terrain. Most of the homes were built between 1918 and 1928 and modeled after the Tuscan villages that so enthralled its developer, Hobart Johnstone Whitley. One of his unique touches was to sink power and telephone lines underground to preserve the views. Gloria Swanson, Charlie Chaplin, and

W. C. Fields were some of its more notable residents.

Remain on Milner until it reaches a T-intersection with Whitley Terrace. Turn left on Whitley, passing Wedgewood Place. Rudolph Valentino liked to walk his two mastiffs down this street. Housewives were known to shoo their husbands off to work so they could be seen watering their gardens out front whenever the Italian heartthrob walked by.

Stay on Whitley Terrace as it skirts the ivy-covered wall for the Hollywood Freeway (US 101) to your left. Though the freeway sliced out the middle of the Heights like a wedge of cake in 1948, it otherwise hasn't changed much thanks to the historic status that preserves its original character. **Just past this freeway wall, follow the street as it jogs south and becomes Whitley Avenue.** Keep an eye out for the house at 2015 Whitley—the former address of Jean Harlow.

Continue on Whitley Avenue until it makes a sharp left and heads back to the lowlands of Franklin Avenue. **Turn right on Franklin, then left on Highland,** proceeding 800 more steps to your starting point near Hollywood & Highland.

If the tourists only knew what they were missing . . .

16
HOLLYWOOD SIGN
A BACKSTAGE PASS

Like the industry it stands for, there's more to the Hollywood Sign than meets the eye. This walk gets you as close to the landmark as is legally possible, with the added bonus of offering the best 360-degree view of Los Angeles. Now, if only that pool was still around . . .

- **TERRAIN:** Hilly
- **SURFACE:** Paved and unpaved
- **FIDO FRIENDLY?:** Yes
- **PARKING:** Street parking near the intersection of Canyon Lake Drive and Innsdale Drive, just north of Lake Hollywood Park at 3200 Canyon Lake Drive, Hollywood

For decades, the Hollywood Sign was a magnet for merry pranksters. From the 1970s through the '90s, its letters were occasionally altered to read different words, like Hollyweed, Holywood, and Ollywood (in protest of the Oliver North Iran-Contra scandal). Others were simply drawn to the idea of touching the sign, feeling its bigness up close. I once hiked up its hillside and was surprised at the abundance of graffiti on the letters that, thankfully, could not be seen from a distance. Because of stunts like these, a security system rivaling Fort Knox was put up, stifling most attempts to access the sign.

In the twenty-first century, a new problem has arisen: the advent of GPS navigation. Rental cars and tourist vans regularly clog the winding streets below the sign, angering Hollywoodland homeowners. Fortunately, *you* are logging

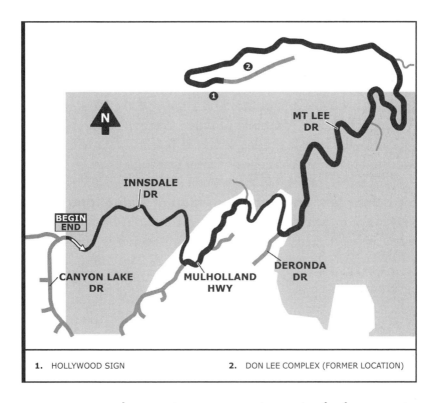

1. HOLLYWOOD SIGN
2. DON LEE COMPLEX (FORMER LOCATION)

10,000 steps today, putting your starting point farther away in the subdued neighborhood of Lake Hollywood Estates, with views that will be closer, safer and more unique than anything the closest public street can offer motorists.

Start by walking to the dead-end of Canyon Lake Drive (Google Maps actually identifies the last 100 feet as Innsdale Drive). **Proceed around the white gate. For the next 800 steps, you'll hike up a gently sloping fire road.** Crane your neck skywards to see red-tailed hawks catching thermals. Meanwhile, on your left, looking up at the Hollywood Sign will give you a really good sense of just how massive it really is.

After bending south, the trail narrows and appears to turn into a private driveway. Rest assured that this is still a public route. A few dozen steps later and you're back on a concrete road. **Turn left on this road, Mulholland Highway,** watching out for cars as there is no sidewalk. Years ago, when Mulholland Drive was built across the Santa Monica Mountains, plans were to continue it past Cahuenga Pass. In fact, the street that goes over Mulholland Dam at Lake Hollywood is technically part of Mulholland Drive. Note the odd engineering here—the road is graded at two different levels, with a rock wall separating the upper and lower portions.

After 400 feet, the median ends and reaches a fork in the road. **Bear left, onto a continuation of Mulholland Highway.** A sign warns, "No Access to the Hollywood Sign!" A rebel at heart, you blaze past the sign, which is actually intended for would-be hikers up the hillside. Two hundred steps later, Mulholland turns into a dirt road. When the Great Depression hit, it was a blessing in disguise for hikers. Money ran out to continue Mulholland into Griffith Park, leaving behind a nice wide fire road instead.

The dirt portion lasts a few hundred feet before turning into blacktop again. Eventually, you'll come to a wrought iron gate barring vehicles from Deronda Drive. To the left of the gate is a pedestrian entryway, next to a white stucco wall. **Walk through the entryway to access Mount Lee Drive,** closed to all traffic except service vehicles. Pause to take in the stunning view of the L.A. skyline. The bluff to your right is a prized spot for fashion shoots, television commercials, and bad music videos.

Continue on Mount Lee Drive for 1,000 steps, at which point a dirt road veers to your right. This is another unpaved section of Mulholland Highway, which heads toward the Griffith Park Observatory. **Continue straight on the paved road,** which begins a pretty steep incline. No whining! Good things come to those who pant.

After another 600 steps, the road bends around the backside of Mount Lee and the view switches to that of the San Fernando Valley, with the Forest Lawn Hollywood Hills Cemetery

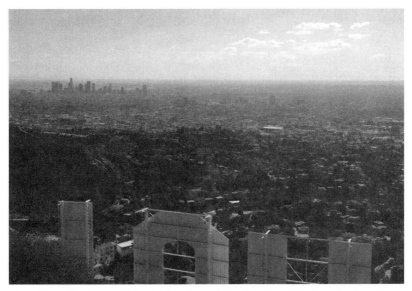

Though less glamorous, the back side of the Hollywood Sign offers its own rewards.

directly below. Proceed another 1,000 steps along the road. As it curves around the crest of Mount Lee, the Los Angeles basin reappears. Suddenly, through a chain-link fence, you see it: the backside of the Hollywood Sign.

It's not until you are standing directly behind the sign that its size can really be appreciated. The original letters from 1923 were five feet taller than the current forty-five-foot ones. Of course, that was back when they spelled out "Hollywoodland." Eventually they fell into disrepair, and the "land" part was never rebuilt. The sign was declared a Historic-Cultural Monument in 1973 and is maintained by the Hollywood Sign Trust. Note the elaborate security system, which includes motion sensors, night-vision cameras, and bullhorns that blast out warnings to trespassers in several different languages.

Just past the sign, Mount Lee Drive terminates at a fence. On the other side is a 300-foot radio tower and a series of buildings that used to belong to Don Lee, a car-dealer-turned-television pioneer who used to broadcast from this perch ("Highest television location in the world!" trumpeted the California Chamber of Commerce). Besides his transmission tower, Lee's complex included a studio and—in true Hollywood fashion—a swimming pool. How great would a refreshing dip feel about now? By the 1950s, the party was over. With the Cold War on everyone's minds, the city took over the site and converted it into a regional control center as part of the Civil Defense network.

STEPPING BACK

On September 16, 1932, twenty-four-year-old Peg Entwistle committed suicide by jumping off the sign's original giant H. Newspapers attributed her demise to despondency over her struggling career as an actress. In a sadly ironic twist, a letter arrived the day she died from the Beverly Hills Playhouse, offering her the starring role in a new play. Her character? A woman who commits suicide by the play's end.

To the left of the fence at the end of Mount Lee Drive, continue on the dirt path that climbs a few steps to the

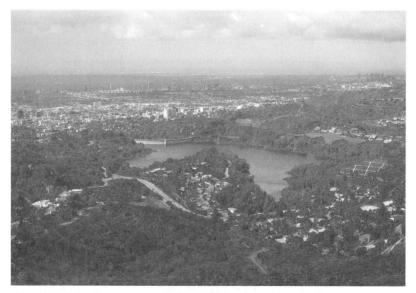

Taking in Lake Hollywood and L.A.'s Westside from Mount Lee.

top of Mount Lee itself.
At 1,709 feet, the 360-de-
gree view is without question the best in Los Ange-

PICNIC OP

The summit of Mount Lee, at the
terminus of Mount Lee Drive.

les. On a clear day, you can see forever . . . or at least to Catalina
Island. To the east, Mount San Jacinto can often be spotted
some ninety miles away. Closer by, Lake Hollywood's sapphire
waters glint in the sunlight, while the Valley side affords views
of the Verdugo and San Gabriel Mountains, which are particularly striking after a snowfall.

Now that you've gone behind the sign's steel curtain, it's
time to rejoin the audience of millions below you. As you **retrace your steps back,** the voice of Norma Desmond rings
in your head. The sign will always be big . . . it's only the real
world that appears small.

17

HOLLYWOOD HILLS

HOORAY FOR LAKE HOLLYWOOD

You don't have to go to the flats of Hollywood to experience the wild life. Simply head to Lake Hollywood—a shimmering blue diamond amidst woodsy pines and oak trees mere minutes from Hollywood and Vine.

- ■ **TERRAIN:** Flat with a short, steep incline
- ■ **SURFACE:** Paved
- ■ **FIDO FRIENDLY?:** No (not allowed at Lake Hollywood)
- ■ **PARKING:** Street parking next to Lake Hollywood Park at 3200 Canyon Lake Drive, Hollywood; from there, walk uphill to the junction of Canyon Lake Drive and Mulholland Highway

This walk starts, as so many things do in Los Angeles, with a gangster and a celebrity. Blessed with an expansive view of Lake Hollywood, Castillo del Lago—"Castle of the Lake"—once hosted an illegal casino run by tenant Benjamin "Bugsy" Siegel, the most feared and influential underworld kingpin in the City of Angels. Years later, pop diva Madonna moved in, slathering the mansion's long retaining wall in stripes of yellow and blood red to the annoyance of neighbors.

We'll get a better glimpse of this palace later in the walk, but for now you can spy the now-white wall at your point of origin. **Begin your walk on an unmarked roadway that starts where Mulholland Highway turns into Canyon**

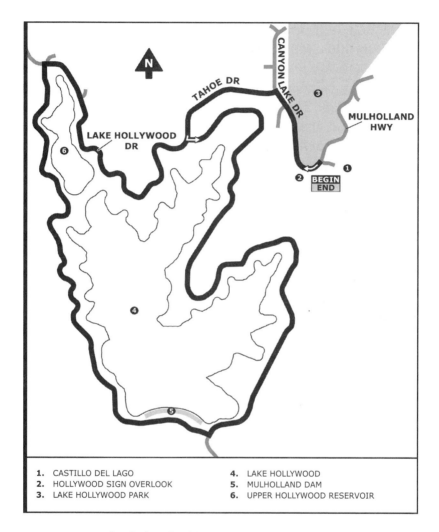

1. CASTILLO DEL LAGO
2. HOLLYWOOD SIGN OVERLOOK
3. LAKE HOLLYWOOD PARK
4. LAKE HOLLYWOOD
5. MULHOLLAND DAM
6. UPPER HOLLYWOOD RESERVOIR

Lake Drive (look for the blue Canyon Lake Drive street sign that reads "3000 N"). Just west of the roadway is an overlook that serves as a popular spot for tourists looking for that money shot of the Hollywood Sign or the L.A. basin.

From the overlook, proceed downhill on Canyon Lake Drive. To your right is Lake Hollywood Park. Canine-loving locals use its large grass field as an unofficial dog park; you use it as the foreground for an Instagram-worthy selfie of the

Hollywood Sign, propped over your shoulder on Mount Lee.

After 400 steps, turn left on Tahoe Drive. Saunter through Lake Hollywood Estates, a pleasant two-block stretch of mid-century homes. When you reach the intersection of Lake Hollywood Drive, you'll get your first view of the chainlink fence that encircles Lake Hollywood.

Turn left to find a pedestrian gate. Enter the road that circumnavigates the reservoir, a popular route for walkers, bicyclists, and out-of-breath, baby-stroller-pushing mommy-runners. A posted sign breaks down the distances around the lake. You're going to do a complete loop—3.3 miles, or about 6,600 steps.

The first 600 steps are your best chance to observe wildlife. Families of deer regularly feast on the hillside foliage to the left. Through the fence to the right, I've seen owls, coyotes, even a gray fox—the only fox I've ever seen in the Santa Monica Mountains—all benefitting from the buffet of vegetation and water within easy reach. You may also encounter wild

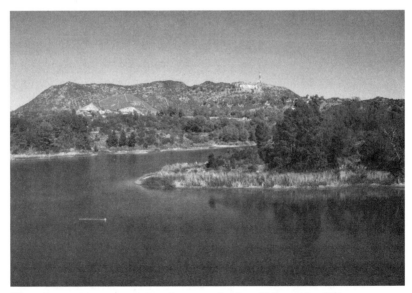

These shimmering waters are less than two miles from Hollywood and Vine.

ducks waddling through moss-laden pools of water that collect on the roadway. Inhale deeply. Appreciate the pine-scented air. If you close your eyes, you could swear you were in the alpines of Big Bear.

After this stretch, the road edges closer to the lake's shoreline, its azure waters fully coming into view. While the reservoir used to provide drinking water for Los Angeles, it has since been taken off-line by the Department of Water and Power. It currently holds less than half of its original capacity of 2.5 billion gallons, but is still impressive enough.

At the halfway point of the perimeter road, you'll find yourself standing on the concrete-arched Mulholland Dam, a Historic-Cultural Monument. You'd be hard-pressed to find a more picturesque vista in the Santa Monica Mountains than the one looking north over the tree-lined lake. This is also a good vantage spot for Castillo del Lago. Its Romanesque tower reigns over the water with the authority of a lighthouse, anchoring the mesa to its east.

STEPPING BACK

As befitting so many early twentieth-century man-made wonders, city boosters turned hyperbolic when heralding the dam's safety, claiming that if Lake Hollywood were "filled with molten lead instead of water, the Dam would still stand." While that sounds like a great ratings-driven TV stunt, water is obviously nothing to scoff at either. Just two years later, the Mulholland-designed Saint Francis Dam near Santa Clarita—which Mulholland Dam was patterned after—burst in the dead of night, claiming 500 lives and ruining the man once hailed a savior.

If the dam looks familiar, that's because it appears in several movies. It famously burst and flooded Hollywood in the 1970s Sensurround cheesefest *Earthquake*, and was the site where Psychopath No. 1 blows two heads off in 2012's *Seven Psychopaths*. Speaking of heads, lean over the railing of the dam's southern face to spot the row of concrete bear heads in

a nod to our state's bear
flag. On the dam's west
end is a dedicatory in-

PICNIC OP
Mulholland Dam, Lake Hollywood.

scription with elegant typeface from 1924.

After passing over Mulholland Dam, proceed 1,200 steps to another dam that separates Lake Hollywood from its smaller counterpart, Upper Hollywood Reservoir. Listen for the sound of rushing water. Peer through the fence and locate its source in the form of a massive drain, like what you'd find in a giant's bathtub. On the far shore is an intake tower. Its lampposted bridge ends in a rotunda and provides a nice visual accent for the lesser lake. If you take this walk in the winter months, your view will be nicely framed by wild toyon clinging to the fence. It's been said that the red, holly-like berry plant—also known as Christmas berry—was the inspiration for the name "Hollywood."

Three hundred steps later, the pedestrian-only perimeter road ends. **Turn right on Lake Hollywood Drive, watching**

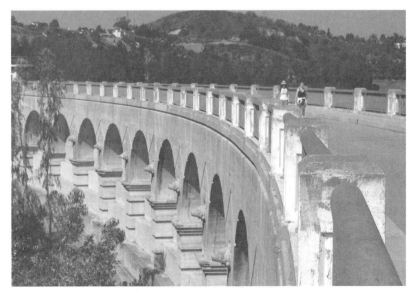

Concrete bear heads adorn Mulholland Dam's arches.

for vehicles. Cross over to the walkway on the north side of the road and complete the 3.3-mile loop by walking the final 1,400 steps to the intersection of Tahoe Drive.

Turn left on Tahoe and walk the 1,000 steps back up to your car. Before decamping, a starry-eyed European couple asks you to take their picture in front of the Hollywood Sign, and perhaps another with the lake in the background. Why not? You already got your own selfie and 10,000 steps to boot.

18

MIRACLE MILE

TREADING ABOVE THE GOO

This walk goes the extra mile—several, actually—as we retrace the natural and man-made wonders of the mid-Wilshire district. And while several icons aren't here anymore, the real miracle is that the best of them still is.

■ **TERRAIN:** Flat
■ **SURFACE:** Mostly paved
■ **FIDO FRIENDLY?:** Yes, assuming no visits to the museums
■ **PARKING:** Street parking or Page Museum lot, on the southwest corner of Curson Avenue and 6th Street, Los Angeles

No other place in Los Angeles is more associated with doomsday than the La Brea Tar Pits. Its grieving family of trapped mammoths serves as a maladroit memento that the primordial goo showed no mercy for any of the 465 species of Pleistocene animals it swallowed up, accounting for more than one million fossils since excavation began in 1906. The asphalt inferno is also where a volcano engulfed Los Angeles in the movie *Volcano*, and was a key locale in the nuclear war film *Miracle Mile*. So what better place to start our walk—and celebrate merely being alive—than the Tar Pits themselves?

Actually, because we sing the songs of the unsung on these walks, **our starting point is a series of rogue tar pools on the southwest corner of 6th Street and Curson Avenue.** Spot them in the grass just north of the parking lot for

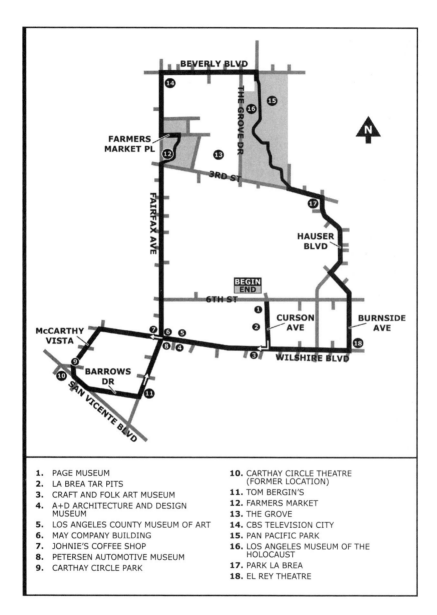

1. PAGE MUSEUM
2. LA BREA TAR PITS
3. CRAFT AND FOLK ART MUSEUM
4. A+D ARCHITECTURE AND DESIGN MUSEUM
5. LOS ANGELES COUNTY MUSEUM OF ART
6. MAY COMPANY BUILDING
7. JOHNIE'S COFFEE SHOP
8. PETERSEN AUTOMOTIVE MUSEUM
9. CARTHAY CIRCLE PARK
10. CARTHAY CIRCLE THEATRE (FORMER LOCATION)
11. TOM BERGIN'S
12. FARMERS MARKET
13. THE GROVE
14. CBS TELEVISION CITY
15. PAN PACIFIC PARK
16. LOS ANGELES MUSEUM OF THE HOLOCAUST
17. PARK LA BREA
18. EL REY THEATRE

the George C. Page Museum. Most of these sludgy puddles are cordoned off, but new ones bubble up all the time, reminders that Hancock Park sits above a giant subterranean oil field that occasionally seeps to the surface. Earlier settlers used the

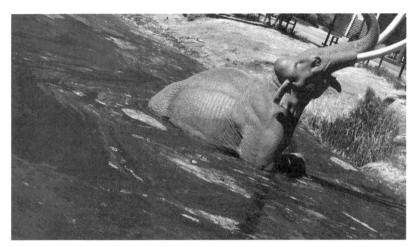

A little help, please? This bellowing mama mammoth has been stuck in the Tar Pits since 1968.

tar to waterproof canoes, baskets, and roofs. I once worked in a nearby office tower where it bled through the walls of an underground parking garage and was hauled off in large barrels.

The area is also known for its high concentration of methane gas, which causes the bubbles in the tar. **As you head south on Curson, stop at Wilshire** and look across the street. On the southwest corner, next to a streetlight, is an adjacent lamppost that appears to have been beheaded. This is actually a vent pipe to release underground methane.

Stick to the north sidewalk as you plod west on Wilshire, which offers the best vantage point of the main tar pit to your right. This stretch is the beginning of Museum Row, which includes the Page, the A+D Architecture and Design Museum, the Craft and Folk Art Museum, the Los Angeles County Museum of Art, and the new Academy of Motion Picture Arts and Sciences Museum.

Unless you feel like logging several thousand more steps, the collections within the museum walls will have to wait for another day. You do, however, have time to photobomb a wedding photo session. Just past the tar pits, the entrance to LACMA is marked by 202 vintage street lamps. Since its unveiling in 2008, the *Urban Light* installation has become one of the most popular picture spots in the city.

STEPPING BACK

Wilshire wasn't just the first grand boulevard in Los Angeles. It was also the first street in the United States to include dedicated left-turn lanes and timed traffic lights—additions that made it clear that streetcars were not welcome!

Continue to the intersection of Wilshire and Fairfax Avenue, which contains three notable landmarks. On the northeast corner is the former May Company department store building, which is dominated by a giant gold column. (Is this what Art Deco on steroids looks like?) Across the street is the former Johnie's coffee shop. Built in 1956, it's one of the last remaining examples of Googie architecture.

Cross over to the southeast corner of the Wilshire/Fairfax intersection. The building here was designed by Welton Becket, whose mid-century icons punctuate the L.A. skyline: the Cinerama Dome, the Capitol Records Building, and the Los Angeles Music Center, to name a few. Opened as a department store in 1962, it became the Petersen Automotive Museum in 1994. Three years later, the museum hosted a music party, after which rapper The Notorious B.I.G. was shot and killed out front. The case remains unsolved.

Hmmm . . . let's flashback to a happier moment. **Continue west for one block on Wilshire, then turn left on McCarthy Vista,** whose grassy median is a vestigial "green carpet" that once led to one of L.A.'s grandest movie palaces. Picture this: It's December 21, 1937, and you are lining the streets along with 30,000 excited onlookers hoping to catch a glimpse of Ginger Rogers, Cary Grant, Marlene Dietrich—and Walt Disney. The glitterati are attending the premiere of Disney's *Snow White and the Seven Dwarfs* at the Carthay Circle Theatre. For the occasion, Disney has converted much of the street into a miniature village called Dwarfland, replete with cottages, a waterwheel, a mini-forest, and appearances by the dwarfs themselves. There's Shirley Temple locking arms with Grumpy, though even her irrepressible charm can't seem to melt his angry heart.

Continue south to Carthay Circle Park, at McCarthy Vista and San Vicente Boulevard. It once held ponds and fountains that framed the entrance to the theater. These days, Dan the Miner—a 1925 bronze statue—is all that's left from that time, though even he disappeared for a while. Several years ago, poor Dan was stolen by two thieves who tried to sell him to a scrap yard before detectives rescued him from a sure molten meltdown.

Across the street are two office buildings. The left one sits at 6310 San Vicente. Behind it is a larger building in the footprint of the former Carthay Circle Theatre, a 1926 Spanish Colonial Revival gem with an octagonal bell tower. Though it was torn down in 1969, the Disney folks never forgot how important it was for the premiere of *Snow White*—both the first feature-length cartoon and the highest-grossing movie of its time. A large-sized reproduction of the theater resides at Disney California Adventure, housing a restaurant.

From McCarthy Vista, turn left on San Vicente, then left on Barrows Drive, which hits Fairfax. Across the street, at 840 Fairfax, spot the neon shamrock sign for Tom Bergin's, which has been serving up Irish coffee since 1936. It claims to have the second-oldest liquor license in Los Angeles County (the Golden Gopher in downtown reportedly has the city's oldest).

From Barrows, stride 1,600 steps north on Fairfax. Cross over to the iconic "Meet me at 3rd and Fairfax" sign on the northeast corner of (what else?) 3rd Street and Fairfax. This corner marks the entrance to the Farmers Market, a boisterous bazaar of 100 shops, restaurants, and produce stalls. In a city of so much change, it's truly a miracle that the market itself has pretty much kept its original layout since opening in 1934. Food options here are a dizzying array of diversity that would make Benetton models proud. After getting your food, find a table and have a seat in one of the market's rickety lime-green folding chairs. Don't forget to visit Bob's Donuts or Bennett's Ice Cream for dessert!

Exit the Farmers Market at its northern edge. A kiosk next to the parking lot provides a pictorial history of this entire block of Fairfax—a nice primer for the next section of this walk.

Leave the parking lot through Farmers Market Place. Turn right on Fairfax, then right on Beverly Boulevard. On your right is CBS Television City, which cranked out classic sitcoms like *All in the Family* and *Three's Company* and timeless game shows like *The Price Is Right*. During a third-grade field trip, I witnessed David Bowie performing on *The Dinah Shore Show* here and seriously thought he was a space alien. Before CBS moved in, this corner held Gilmore Stadium and Gilmore Field, where the Hollywood Stars minor league baseball team played. However, after the Dodgers migrated from Brooklyn in 1958, the team became irrelevant overnight. It relocated to Salt Lake City and Gilmore Field was torn down.

Proceed 800 steps on Beverly—past the post office—until you reach Curson Avenue. Turn right into the parking lot for Pan Pacific Park. Immediately to your left is the park's recreation center. Its crested green tower is a nod to the Pan Pacific Auditorium, a Streamline Moderne jewel from 1937 that burned down in 1989. Like the Petersen Museum, it was designed by Welton Becket. And, just as they did with the

SIDE-STEP

If you'd prefer to walk through The Grove—Rick J. Caruso's Disneyfied version of a main street retail district—head directly east of the Farmers Market. The mall sits on the site of the former Gilmore Drive-In. Rejoin the book's route by turning left at The Grove Drive, then right on Beverly Boulevard.

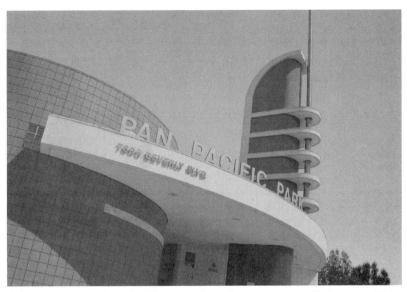

The Streamline Moderne pylon of Pan Pacific Park's rec center recalls the original four towers of Pan Pacific Auditorium.

Carthay Circle Theatre, the Disney folks recreated the lost relic at Disney California Adventure, incorporating its famous four-towered façade into the park's entrance.

South of the parking lot, follow the walking trails into the park, which is also home to the underrated Los Angeles Museum of the Holocaust. Much of the museum is integrated into the terraced landscape of the park.

The park extends about two blocks, letting out on 3rd Street near a bust of an influential

STEPPING BACK

This route includes the footprints of two of my personal "Top Five Dearly Departed Landmarks in L.A." Besides the Carthay Circle Theatre and Pan Pacific Auditorium, it's a travesty that these three architectural masterpieces are not still around for us to appreciate: the Ambassador Hotel in mid-Wilshire, downtown's Richfield Building, and NBC's West Coast Radio City Studios at Hollywood and Sunset.

Jewish American patriot named Haym Salomon. **Head east on 3rd to Hauser Boulevard and**

PICNIC OP
Pan Pacific Park, 7600 Beverly Boulevard.

turn right. To your right is a clutch of boxy residential towers from 1948 known as Park La Brea. Can you think of any other housing complex that so divides Angelenos? People seem to either love it or hate it. To me, it looks uncomfortably similar to drab communist-era flats I've seen in Eastern Europe, even with the colorful paint job designed to cover up its original eggshell walls.

Exit Park La Brea by turning left on Burnside Avenue and walking until you hit Wilshire. Two stores east of the corner, at 5515 Wilshire, is the Art Deco-influenced El Rey Theatre. On the south side of Wilshire, covering one entire block and eleven stories, is the former Desmond's department store. When it opened in 1929, Desmond's catered to our burgeoning love affair with the automobile by putting the parking lot and main entrance in the back. Such was the Miracle Mile concept, as laid out by real estate developer A. W. Ross.

Continue west on Wilshire until you reach Curson. Before you turn right to head back to your car, cross over to the traffic island. There, in the middle of the street, is a sculpture of Mr. Ross himself—a fitting end to our "miraculous" walk. An epitaph reads: "A. W. Ross, founder and developer of the Miracle Mile. Vision to see, wisdom to know, courage to do." Only in Los Angeles would we celebrate someone for contributing to our choking traffic!

19

WILSHIRE CENTER

A FEW MIRACLES OF ITS OWN

Though its name isn't as catchy as the Miracle Mile, Wilshire Center was once the epicenter of celebrity cool before the Westside pushed farther west. But the past is still very much present on this eclectic route that includes Koreatown and MacArthur Park.

- **TERRAIN:** Flat
- **SURFACE:** Mostly paved
- **FIDO FRIENDLY?:** Yes
- **PARKING:** Street parking near the corner of Wilshire Boulevard and Wilton Place, Los Angeles

Wilshire Boulevard bears the name of its developer, but in reality Gaylord Wilshire laid out only a few blocks of Los Angeles's first grand street. Subdividing acres of barley fields in 1896, Wilshire built one of the city's first fashionable residential districts in the Westlake district. Westward sprawl quickly followed, leaving a legacy of buildings that have become timeless classics.

Start at the southwest corner of Wilton Place and Wilshire. Head west several paces to the house at 4016 Wilshire. Built in 1918, it's reportedly the last house standing

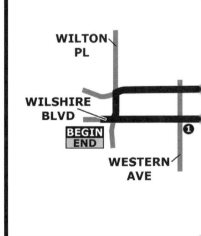

on the entire boulevard, which extends all the way to the beach! Much respect, homie.

Turn around and head east on Wilshire. At Wilton, Korean signage will start to appear as you reach the western

> ### STEPPING BACK
>
> Wilton is also the start-point for a "Miracle Mile" of a different sort. There are literally hundreds of religious congregations in Wilshire Center spread across all faiths. Many of the ornate temples and churches along Wilshire are approaching the century mark.

boundary of Koreatown. Roughly three square miles, K-Town is a late-comer compared to other East Asian enclaves like Chinatown and Little Tokyo. But its nightlife trumps even Hollywood's, with the highest concentration of restaurants and bars in L.A. It's also the city's most faddish district—businesses pop up as quickly as they disappear, and discovering what's new is part of the fun.

1. WILTERN THEATER
2. WILSHIRE BOULEVARD TEMPLE
3. ROBERT F. KENNEDY INSPIRATION PARK
4. ROBERT F. KENNEDY COMMUNITY SCHOOLS
5. BROWN DERBY (FORMER LOCATION)
6. GAYLORD APARTMENTS
7. BULLOCKS WILSHIRE BUILDING
8. LAFAYETTE PARK
9. MACARTHUR PARK
10. LAKE
11. LANGER'S DELI
12. FIRST CONGREGATIONAL CHURCH
13. CHAPMAN MARKET

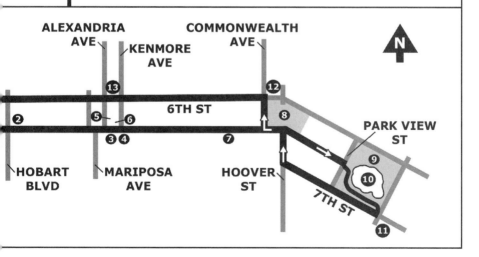

Two blocks later, you'll come to Western Avenue. On the southeast corner is the Wiltern Theater, the 1931 blue-green paean to Art Deco. Shockingly (or perhaps not, this being L.A.), the structure was once threatened with the wrecking ball. It has since been refurbished, given historic status, and is a great place to catch a concert. Los Angeles, incidentally, is a hybrid-happy city. And I'm not just talking cars. "Wiltern" is a hybrid of "Wilshire" and "Western." Comb the city and you'll find other corner buildings that have adopted the names of their intersecting streets, like Silversun Liquor (Silver Lake and Sunset Boulevards), Norwood Market (Normandie Avenue and Hollywood Boulevard) and the girlie-sounding Rox-San Medical Building in Beverly Hills (Roxbury Drive and Santa Monica Boulevard).

In another 400 steps, you'll come to the Wilshire Boulevard Temple, on the corner of Hobart Boulevard. The oldest synagogue in Los Angeles is capped by a massive Byzantine dome that's visible from Griffith Park. Inside are biblical murals commissioned by Warner Bros. head honcho Jack Warner in 1929. Louis B. Mayer, Irving Thalberg, and Carl Laemmle were just a few of the other Hollywood moguls who worshipped here on High Holidays during filmdom's Golden Age.

Proceed another four blocks to the twin ghosts of Important Things Past. Just past Mariposa Avenue on the right side is the former site of the Ambassador Hotel, whose razing remains one of the bitterest defeats for preservationists. Its Cocoanut Grove nightclub drew top-drawer musical talent like Louis Armstrong, Judy Garland, and Frank Sinatra. Beyond the frivolity, the Ambassador was where presidential hopeful Robert Kennedy was assassinated in 1968. Robert F. Kennedy Inspiration Park, a tasteful memorial to RFK, lines Wilshire Boulevard. The former hotel site is now the location of the Robert F. Kennedy Community Schools, which is better than what *could* have gone here, had prospective buyer Donald Trump had his way: the world's tallest skyscraper, no doubt with his name emblazoned in lights across the night sky.

Across the street abutting Alexandria Avenue is a ghastly stucco strip mall once occupied by the original Brown Derby restaurant. The legendary Hollywood hangout was outfitted in a giant brown hat, its walls festooned with caricatures of its famous customers. Look toward the back of the mini-mall and you can make out a round protrusion that looks like a giant egg shell. Yep, that's the original dome that made up the restaurant's hat. Seems a little sacrilegious to me, though I suppose it's no different than converting old movie palaces into flea markets. Squint hard enough through its curvature and you can make out Groucho Marx forking a Cobb salad, invented in the Derby's kitchen.

Just east of the mini-mall, at 3355 Wilshire, is the historic Gaylord Apartments. The ground floor is occupied by the HMS Bounty, a nautical-themed restaurant that once fed Sir Winston Churchill. The lobby next to the restaurant contains a nice collection of photos and artifacts of this building and

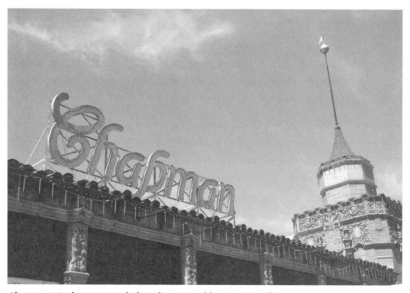

Chapman Market is regarded as the city's oldest mini-mall.

nearby apartment high-rises. Their elegance is matched by their names: the Asbury, the Langham, the Piccadilly, and the Fox Normandie, many of which still have neon signs on their roofs.

Continuing east brings you to another Art Deco classic at 3050. Built in 1929 by Donald Parkinson—the same architect who helped design City Hall and Union Station—the Bullocks Wilshire department store was known as a "cathedral of commerce." It has since been repurposed as a bastion for barristers, housing the Southwestern Law School. A few hundred steps later, Wilshire curves and enters the Westlake area. After passing Lafayette Park, you'll come to the more famous MacArthur Park several blocks later. The same park that is "melting in the dark" in the famous disco song, MacArthur Park has an artificial lake that is the direct descendant of a natural spring. Like this entire area, the park itself—a Historic-Cultural Monument—is on an upswing.

Enter MacArthur Park at the southeast corner of Wilshire and Park View Street, where a 1920 statue of former *Los Angeles Times* publisher Harrison Gray Otis stands sentry alongside that of a newsboy hollering "Extra! Extra!" (What else would he be saying?) The statues make cameos in Buster Keaton and Charlie Chaplin shorts. **Stroll the park on a southerly route** to find other sculptures, some of them hidden behind overgrown shrubs.

Exit MacArthur Park at its southeast corner. Catty-corner from the park is Langer's Deli, founded in 1947 when the neighborhood was decidedly different. Hope you brought your appetite—you'll need it as you slip into a booth and order up a hot pastrami sandwich on double-baked rye bread. Many swear by the #19 (a pastrami and cole slaw sandwich), but you can't miss with any of their culinary creations!

PICNIC OP

Lakeside at MacArthur Park, 2230 6th Street.

Leaving Langer's, head west on 7th Street. Turn right on Hoover, left on Wilshire, then right on Commonwealth Avenue. On the northeast corner of 6th Street and Commonwealth is the First Congregational Church, which boasts the world's largest pipe organ.

Continue west on 6th, a retail route through Koreatown that offers infinite boba and frozen dessert concoctions. Architecturally, the 1929 Chapman Market building is a must-see—it takes up the entire block after Kenmore Avenue. The elaborate decorative details of its Churrigueresque façade trace their roots to seventeenth-century Spain. It also holds the distinction as the world's first drive-in market, with a short tunnel off Kenmore leading to a parking lot. Step on the south side of 6th to observe the rusty "Chapman Market" sign perched on the red-tile roof.

From there, it's 2,000 more steps back to your starting point at Wilton, near Wilshire. Good thing for you, the Snow-LA Shavery is across the street from Chapman. A refreshing Black Sesame Snow with fresh fruit and condensed milk should last for much of the way back.

20

GREATER HANCOCK PARK

THE PLATINUM SQUARE

The Westside may have the Platinum Triangle (Beverly Hills, Holmby Hills, and Bel-Air), but Mid-City has it beat, both in age and geometry. I call it the Platinum Square, a ritzy route of generous lawns, concealed creeks, and a little bit of magic.

- **TERRAIN:** Flat
- **SURFACE:** Paved
- **FIDO FRIENDLY?:** Yes
- **PARKING:** Street parking near the intersection of Beverly Boulevard and Larchmont Boulevard; lots in Larchmont Village

Hancock Park is often invoked by Angelenos the same way we use West L.A. to describe any Westside community from Palms to Mar Vista to, well, West L.A. While there *is* a neighborhood of Hancock Park, its broader region includes Windsor Square, Fremont Place, and Brookside, four points on a geographic quadrant that make up some of the oldest and most prestigious real estate in Los Angeles.

From Beverly Boulevard, head south on Larchmont Boulevard through Larchmont Village, a three-block business district with a small-town feel that is feverishly protected by local residents. Businesses include specialty shops, indie book stores, a confectionary, and a general store called Landis that dates back to the 1920s.

PICNIC OP

Benches along Larchmont Boulevard in Larchmont Village.

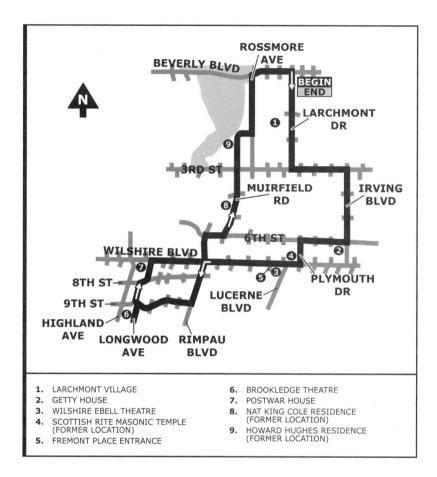

1. LARCHMONT VILLAGE
2. GETTY HOUSE
3. WILSHIRE EBELL THEATRE
4. SCOTTISH RITE MASONIC TEMPLE
   (FORMER LOCATION)
5. FREMONT PLACE ENTRANCE
6. BROOKLEDGE THEATRE
7. POSTWAR HOUSE
8. NAT KING COLE RESIDENCE
   (FORMER LOCATION)
9. HOWARD HUGHES RESIDENCE
   (FORMER LOCATION)

Larchmont also corners the market on charming sidewalk bistros. Since this walk does not pass by any other restaurants, this is the time to chow down!

One thousand steps from Beverly Boulevard, go left on 3rd Street, entering the residential portion of Windsor Square. Turn right on Irving Boulevard, one of several streets given stuffy British names by their developer, Robert A. Rowan, who set out to capture the aura of the English countryside. Rowan even went so far as to sink all the utility wires underground—unheard of in 1911. All he was lacking was a way to recreate bitterly cold winters.

At the southwest corner of Irving and 6th Street is a Tudor Revival named the Getty House after the son of oil baron J. Paul Getty. Beginning with Tom Bradley, the 1921 manse has been the official residence of Los Angeles mayors, although Antonio Villaraigosa vacated in 2007 when he and his wife separated and she stayed behind with the kids. Some of these houses on Irving are technically the world's most expensive mobile homes. They were moved here from Westlake (MacArthur Park) in the 1920s.

Turn right on 6th, then left on Plymouth Drive. Cross Wilshire Boulevard and turn right. On the corner of Wilshire and Lucerne Boulevard is the Wilshire Ebell Theatre, home to the Ebell Club, a philanthropic women's organization that dates back to 1894. Amelia Earhart made her final speaking appearance here in 1937. Catty-corner is a former Scottish Rite Masonic Temple designed by Millard Sheets, whose renowned mosaics can be found on the old Home Savings and Loan buildings around L.A.

Proceed 400 steps west on Wilshire. On your left is an ornate gateway leading to Fremont Place, a privately owned neighborhood of seventy-three homes built around the same time as Windsor Square. Homeowners included entrepreneurs like King C. Gillette of the Gillette razor company and Bank of America founder A. P. Giannini, though its most famous resident was probably Muhammad Ali. You can't walk its streets unless you live here, but you *can* take a virtual tour of its homes on YouTube, where a realtor has conveniently posted a drive-by video of its impressive mansions while lamenting in voiceover, "L.A. really does not have a lot of gated communities . . . which is a shame."

Hoof it another 500 steps down Wilshire, then go left on Rimpau Boulevard and right on 9th Street. You are now entering Brookside, a little-known neighborhood established in 1979 that is more than just a pretty-sounding name. But first, wanna see some magic? **Turn left on Longwood**

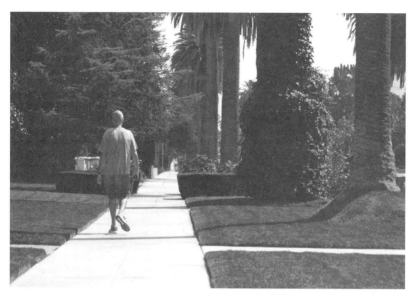

Hancock Park's flat sidewalks, leafy estates, and broad, tidy lawns summon the stroller.

Avenue and press on to a Mission-style job on your right—address 929. It belongs to the Larsen family, founders of Hollywood's Magic Castle. Behind the house is a seventy-seat venue known as the Brookledge Theatre, which has hosted invitation-only magic shows since the 1940s. Orson Welles used to park his considerable frame on a battered old sofa that resides in the room. You can still see magic shows at the Brookledge if you know the secret password. (Pssst . . . the password is: get to know someone in L.A.'s magic community.)

As its name implies, Brookledge is perched on the side of a brook. Many residences in Brookside have a natural creek known as Arroyo de Los Jardines running through their backyards. But like the magic shows at Brookledge, the creek often pulls a disappearing act; it's largely subterranean until it hits Melrose Avenue. After that, it plays peek-a-boo before finally merging with Ballona Creek. Even when it *is* visible, it cuts through some pretty exclusive real estate, like the links of the

Wilshire Country Club, where it can be spied through a fence.

To catch glimpses of brooksides in Brookside, **head north up Longwood and turn right on 8th Street.** Behind the Mission Revival house on your right is a hedge-covered fence along the sidewalk. Peek through the leaves and spot a trickling creek with bridges under the trees. The ar-

> **EXTRA STEPS**
>
> At the fenced-off southeast corner of Wilshire and Highland is a former model home known as the Postwar House—later known as the House of Tomorrow. It was used to entice returning World War II veterans into buying similar homes. It doesn't look like much now, but when it opened in 1946, it featured many elements we now take for granted, like an electric garbage disposal, central air, a big-screen TV, and a remote-controlled garage door opener . . . useful for when you want to park your jetpack.

royo can also be seen from 8th Street's northern sidewalk, behind the white stucco residence on the corner. Look past the clump of trees to the left of the driveway, then make haste so no one thinks you're a peeping Tom!

Proceed north on Longwood, then turn right on Wilshire. Go left on Rimpau, entering the well-heeled domiciles of Hancock Park, which reflect developer G. Allan Hancock's vision of Period Revival homes fronted by broad lawns and set back fifty feet from the street.

After turning right on 6th, hang a left on Muirfield Road. The Tudor Revival at 401 Muirfield used to belong to Nat King Cole. When the black entertainer moved into the predominantly white neighborhood in 1948, it's safe to say that no one brought over a tray of cookies. Hancock Park residents left racial epithets in his yard and harassed his family. A petition circulated the neighborhood to rid it of "undesirables." Ever the cool customer, Nat—who performed nearby at the Cocoanut Grove, where many of his neighbors undoubtedly paid to see his sold-out shows—reportedly deadpanned, "If I see any undesirables, I'll let you know."

If anyone could be considered an undesirable, it might have been Howard Hughes. The playboy billionaire lived in the hacienda at 211 Muirfield behind the ninth hole of the Wilshire Country Club, cycling through a parade of starlet-mistresses before bailing out of the house to avoid paying state income taxes.

From Hughes's old lair, **Muirfield turns and connects with Rossmore Avenue,** the eastern boundary of Hancock Park. **Hang a left on Rossmore, then a right on Beverly Boulevard,** which takes you back to the cozy confines of Larchmont Village.

21

WEST HOLLYWOOD

ROCK WALK

Rock 'n' roll may have been born in Memphis, but from the 1960s through the '80s, no place rocked harder than West Hollywood. Relive those heady times with a club-hopping trip that breaks on through to the other side.

- ■ **TERRAIN:** Flat with stairs and slight inclines
- ■ **SURFACE:** Paved
- ■ **FIDO FRIENDLY?:** Yes
- ■ **PARKING:** Lot adjacent to Barney's Beanery, at 8447 Santa Monica Boulevard, West Hollywood

The history of West Hollywood can be summed up by the original Barney's Beanery, the starting point for this walk. It not only occupies the nexus of two major streets, it also straddles the city's two most dominant subcultures—and not always comfortably. Built as a simple roadside diner in 1920, it became a mecca for the bohemian/rocker crowd by the 1960s. Marlon Brando and Jack Nicholson bopped in for drinks, the Doors played pool into the wee hours, and Janis Joplin was such a frequent guest, she had a preferred booth—number thirty-four.

Concurrently, the city's gay community was growing. Needless to say, a nasty sign above the bar that invoked a gay pejorative ("F****s—Stay Out") did not go over well with many clientele. Despite mass picketing in 1970 to have the sign removed, it lasted until 1984. Since then, however, Barney's has happily changed with the times while otherwise keeping its divey atmosphere. Oh yeah, and they also make a mean bowl

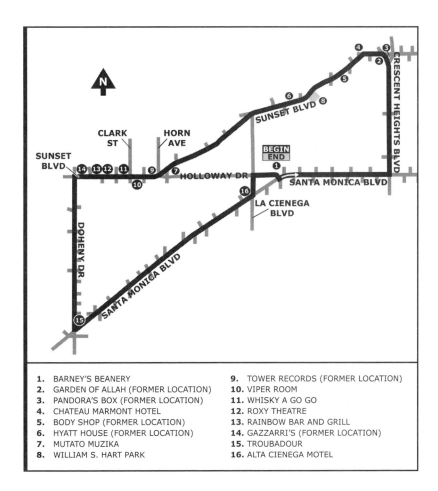

1. BARNEY'S BEANERY
2. GARDEN OF ALLAH (FORMER LOCATION)
3. PANDORA'S BOX (FORMER LOCATION)
4. CHATEAU MARMONT HOTEL
5. BODY SHOP (FORMER LOCATION)
6. HYATT HOUSE (FORMER LOCATION)
7. MUTATO MUZIKA
8. WILLIAM S. HART PARK
9. TOWER RECORDS (FORMER LOCATION)
10. VIPER ROOM
11. WHISKY A GO GO
12. ROXY THEATRE
13. RAINBOW BAR AND GRILL
14. GAZZARRI'S (FORMER LOCATION)
15. TROUBADOUR
16. ALTA CIENEGA MOTEL

of chili. Fuel up here before starting our Rock Walk.

From Barney's Beanery, trek east on Santa Monica Boulevard, then north on Crescent Heights Boulevard. After 2,000 steps, you'll reach Sunset Boulevard. On the southwest corner is an ugly strip mall that bears no resemblance to the earthly paradise it replaced. From the 1920s to 1959, this site was the Garden of Allah, a legendary bungalow hotel where the bacchanalia never ended. Actors like Humphrey Bogart, Greta Garbo, and Errol Flynn mingled with such literati as F. Scott Fitzgerald, Ernest Hemingway, and

Robert Benchley, who once had an accomplice steer him from room to room in a wheelbarrow. His mission: more gin. The swimming pool existed somewhere in the current parking lot that separates a bank from fast-food restaurants. Ponder the sultry image of Marlene Dietrich skinny-dipping after hours. "Sex in America—an obsession," she once complained. "In other parts of the world—a fact."

But where Hollywood's elite preferred to keep their affairs private, not so for the youth of 1966. This same intersection spawned the very public demonstration that inspired the Buffalo Springfield song "For What It's Worth" and the counter-culture flick *Riot on Sunset Strip*. The flashpoint occurred at Pandora's Box, a *very* small club squeezed into a traffic island. Peter Fonda and Jack Nicholson (maybe he had just come from Barney's?) were among the hundreds protesting a recently-enacted curfew against "those darn hippies." Pandora's Box was torn down shortly thereafter, but the island it sat on is still there. Look for the triangular-shaped dirt median to the right of the strip mall, with a

> **STEPPING BACK**
>
> The Strip owes its existence to a quirky zoning law. For decades, it was an unincorporated part of Los Angeles County outside the realm of the LAPD. Burlesque bars, gay brothels, nightclubs, and speakeasies proliferated, setting the template for the good times that continue today.

bus stop and a couple of scrawny palm trees. This intersection also marks the eastern edge of the Sunset Strip, which continues west for a mile and a half before reaching Beverly Hills.

As you **head west on Sunset,** the fabled addresses roll by with regularity. Some of rock 'n' roll's greatest hits include: the Chateau Marmont Hotel at 8221, the Historic-Cultural landmark where Led Zeppelin rode their motorcycles through the lobby and Blues Brother John Belushi died of a drug overdose; the Body Shop at 8250, a former strip club that employed Courtney Love and provided the location for Mötley Crüe's

"Girls, Girls, Girls" video; and the ex-Hyatt House at 8401, which earned the nickname "Riot House" due to the rowdy rockers who trashed the place, most famously when members of the Rolling Stones and the Who hucked TVs from their windows. Alternative music fans will want to pay tribute to Mutato Muzika—the lime-green circular building that looks like a UFO at 8760, recording studio of Mark Mothersbaugh, lead singer and cofounder of Devo.

Of course, as the music business blew up, so did the billboards, resulting in the flashy street-level advertisements along the Strip that are still around today. If you were a band in the 1970s, you had officially arrived when your record company sprang for an ad, which invariably had some mechanical part like moving eyeballs or spouting steam—or female body parts that caused many near-miss accidents.

After 1,200 steps on Sunset, you'll reach Horn Avenue—a symbolic intersection. For decades, the northwest corner currently occupied by Gibson was anchored by Tower Records, a popular music mecca where every new

PICNIC OP

William S. Hart Park—accessible from the Strip. Entrance just before the Sunset Tower Hotel at 8358 Sunset Boulevard.

record release was given the VIP treatment. Tower was more than a store; its brash red-and-yellow decor shouted out that you were now entering the western end of the Strip—the *true* epicenter of rock 'n' roll not just in WeHo, but in the world.

A block past Horn Avenue, at 8852, is the Viper Room. Flowers are occasionally placed in front of the music club, where River Phoenix collapsed and died on the sidewalk on Halloween night, 1993. In its former incarnation as the Melody Room, the club hosted shadowy toughs like Mickey Cohen and Bugsy Siegel.

One more block brings you to the Whisky A Go Go. Lots of rock clubs like to bill themselves as "world famous," but in the Whisky's case, it's actually true. Beginning in 1964, the modest venue on the corner of Sunset and Clark Street hosted legions of legendary live performances, many of them memorialized on records. The Doors were the house band here before they got big. A generation later, I experienced several great punk rock shows here that have never left me (seriously . . . my ears are still ringing from Sonic Youth).

Another two blocks leads you to the Roxy Theatre, at 9009. Despite opening a decade after the Whisky, it quickly equaled its stature. The Roxy also benefitted from its neighbor, the Rainbow Bar and Grill, where it always feels like 2 AM. Step inside and soak up some genuine rock 'n' roll atmosphere—not hard to do since the smell of stale beer and whiskey seems permanently etched into its carpet. If these walls could talk, their stories would rival those of the female servers, who often doubled as groupies. The Rainbow Room, as it's often called, figures prominently in at least one tell-all memoir.

For Axl Rose and Slash, it was a short walk (or stumble)

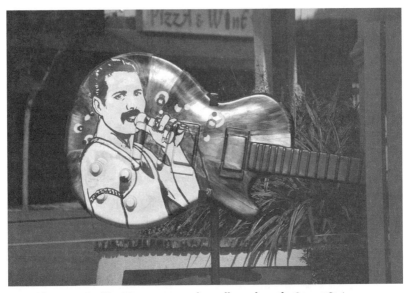

Queen frontman Freddie Mercury serenades walkers along the Sunset Strip.

between the Rainbow and Gazzarri's. Their band, Guns N' Roses, ushered in the hair-band craze of the late 1980s at the former club located at 9039. Gazzarri's most famous graduates were Van Halen, who played their first performance there on April 4, 1974, on their way to world domination. The club closed for good after sustaining damage from the 1994 Northridge Earthquake, though one could argue that the rise of '90s grunge dealt the knockout blow.

A few more steps brings you to Doheny Drive. Time to leave the Strip behind. **Turn left and stride 1,200 steps down Doheny to Santa Monica Boulevard.** On the northeast corner is the Troubadour, the last club of our Rock Walk. One of the cool things about West Hollywood's clubs is their different personalities. The Troubadour came of age in the late 1950s as a coffeehouse that favored more "serious" artists. Not surprisingly, a decade later it launched the careers of singer-songwriters Joni Mitchell, Jackson Browne, and the Eagles.

Head east on Santa Monica, entering the so-called Boys Town, the vibrant commercial stretch of WeHo's gay community. The nicely landscaped median that runs through the middle of the boulevard used to be an eyesore. Up through the 1970s, it was nothing more than a deteriorating gravel bed supporting rusty freight train tracks. To this day, the converted railroad median ends at Barney's Beanery, though the tracks themselves used to extend as far east as Seward Street, where old rails still peek through the pavement.

Upon reaching La Cienega Boulevard, turn left. Just off the corner at 1005 is the Alta Cienega Motel. The Doors had an office here, and Jim Morrison himself lived in room thirty-two. Is it any wonder that he spent seemingly half his waking hours at Barney's Beanery, a mere block away? Retrace the Lizard King's steps and complete your Rock Walk by **turning right on Holloway Drive.**

22

BALDWIN HILLS

FLOOD-AND-FANCY-FREE

Baldwin Hills' past and present go together like oil and water. No, really. This out-and-back route retraces the roles each played in the formation of this affluent mid-city community.

- **TERRAIN:** Mostly flat with one long incline
- **SURFACE:** Paved and unpaved
- **FIDO FRIENDLY?:** Yes
- **PARKING:** Street parking near the intersection of Carmona Avenue and Coliseum Street, Baldwin Hills

Baldwin Hills can be divided into two eras: pre-flood and post-flood. While Jefferson Boulevard serves as its flat, northern boundary, its southern edge used to be defined by a 292-million-gallon reservoir carved into its namesake hills.

But at precisely 3:38 PM on December 14, 1963, everything changed. A rupture in the Baldwin Hills Reservoir's dam sent a fifty-foot wall of water down the hillside. Five people were swept away to their deaths, with 275 homes either damaged or destroyed. Live news footage showed cars being tossed around like Hot Wheels—500 in all. The first part of this walk takes you directly through the flood zone.

From its junction with Carmona Avenue, head east on Coliseum Street along the northern sidewalk. By the way, ever wonder what Coliseum Street is doing here, some five miles west of the *actual* Los Angeles Memorial Coliseum? Baldwin Hills hosted the world's first-ever Olympic

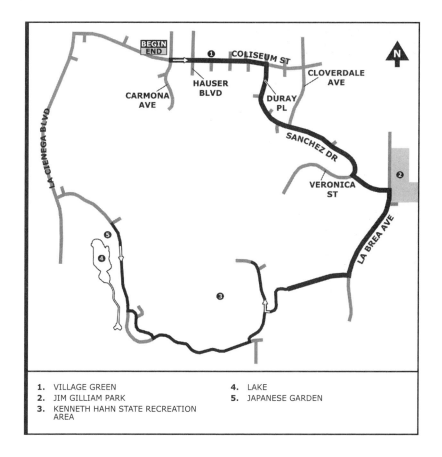

1. VILLAGE GREEN
2. JIM GILLIAM PARK
3. KENNETH HAHN STATE RECREATION AREA
4. LAKE
5. JAPANESE GARDEN

Village during the 1932 Games. Coliseum Street pays tribute to the venerable venue, where several events and ceremonies were held.

In one block—just past Hauser Boulevard on your left—you'll reach the Village Green, a throwback to the 1940s. Initially called Baldwin Hills Village, the National Historic Landmark was considered the height of community planning in its day. Two-story houses fan out from garage courts, which are clustered around a central green over sixty-four acres. The residences (now condos) still look neat and tidy with their horizontal lines and gabled roofs.

Things were anything but neat and tidy when the dam

broke. Lying at the base of the hill, Village Green got pummeled with water, sludge, and detritus. The first court you come across—Court Eight—made the live news when a helicopter tried to pluck trapped residents out of harm's way. Farther down, the dwellings surrounding Courts Six and Seven got socked even harder.

Once you reach Court Six, cross over Duray Place and head south. Duray feeds into picture-perfect streets of mid-century homes. Because of restrictive laws in affluent white communities, Baldwin Hills was one of the first upper-middle-class black neighborhoods in L.A. Famous neighbors included Ike and Tina Turner, Ray Charles, and Mayor Tom Bradley. **Continue as Duray becomes Sanchez Drive.** As the road turns left, you'll pass Cloverdale Avenue. This north-south street bore the worst of the flood, lying directly in the water's angry path.

Continue on Sanchez until it reaches Veronica Street, then turn left. After one short block, you'll hit La Brea Avenue. The park across the street is Jim Gilliam Park, named after the popular Dodger infielder who died suddenly in 1978.

Turn right on La Brea, taking it up a gradual incline. Be mindful to stay off the road—some stretches do not have a sidewalk, requiring you to walk on a well-trod dirt path. **After 600 steps, you'll come across an unmarked paved road to your right.** The chain-link gate is usually locked to cars. Either way, **walk around the gate and walk up the road,** taking a sort of back door to Kenneth Hahn State Recreation Area. Don't be discouraged by the presence of ominous signs—this area has long been used by park-goers accessing the park from La Brea.

As the road narrows and curves to the

SIDE-STEP

If you are dissuaded by the signs, proceed up La Brea another 600 steps. Access the dirt hiking trail that climbs the hillside, just past a pepper tree, and reconnect with this route at the top.

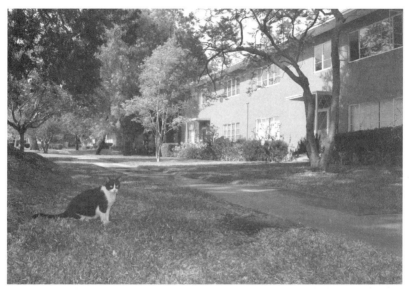

People aren't the only ones who appreciate the Village Green's mid-century charms.

left, you will come to the lip of a large, grassy basin.
You are now standing in the former bowl of the Baldwin Hills
Reservoir. Instead of rebuilding the lake, former L.A. County
supervisor Kenneth Hahn came up with the idea of filling it
in and creating a 308-acre park. The north end of the basin is
where the dam used to be, replaced by a walkway that encircles the old reservoir. **Venture to the northern edge and
look down,** imagining the houses crumbling like sand castles during a high tide as they did on that horrific day. Props
to you, Kenneth!

    **Double back on the pathway that circles the basin
and walk onto the park's main road,** which cuts through
groves of trees as it crawls west. Out in the distance are a sea
of dinosaur-shaped oil jacks, pumping away. The Inglewood
Oil Fields are one of the last active oil bastions in the city and
have appeared in numerous movies. *L.A. Confidential* director Curtis Hanson set a climactic shoot-out in front of them.
What is it about these nodding pumpjacks that makes them so

sinister-looking? Present-
ly, the operators of these
oil deposits have stirred
fracking concerns, but
the pools already courted
controversy once before.
In 1976, federal geologists
ruled that overexploita-
tion of the Inglewood Oil
Fields caused the land under the reservoir's earthen
dam to sink, leading to its
breach.

After you curve to the
right, a man-made stream
will come into view. The
stream has dozens of
strategically placed rocks

STEPPING BACK

Many of the oil wells abut
La Cienega Boulevard. Under
normal circumstances, La Cienega
would provide the quickest way
back to your point of origin, but
pedestrians are forbidden on it. In
addition to a "No Ped" zone, this
stretch of La Cienega has a 55
mph speed limit, a center median,
call boxes, on/off-ramps ... gee,
sounds an awful lot like a freeway.
Wait a minute—it *is* a freeway! The
La Cienega Freeway was
supposed to start in El Segundo
and forge a path into the Valley
as part of Route 170. The two
and a half miles between Slauson
Avenue and Rodeo Road is the
only section that ever got built.

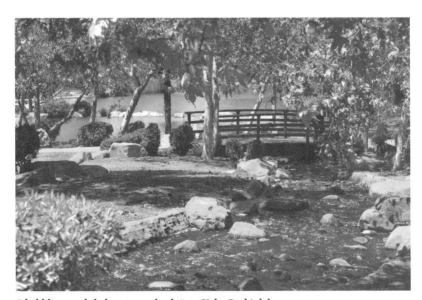

A babbling, rock-laden stream leads into Hahn Park's lake.

that encourage hopping through the water. It leads to a serene lake stocked with fish—truly one of the more overlooked gems in L.A.'s park system. Reclining in the shade of a tree along its grassy shoreline, don't be surprised if you find yourself drifting off into a catnap.

PICNIC OP

Lakeside at the Kenneth Hahn State Recreation Area, 4100 La Cienega Boulevard.

EXTRA STEPS

If you want to push on, the park also has a Japanese Garden and lotus pond, 600 steps north of the lake and past the gatehouse.

Your nap doesn't last long. You are rudely awakened by a goose honking in your ear. If you packed a picnic, he probably wants your food. You've got to get going anyway—at 5,000 steps, the lake is only the halfway point. **Return to your car the way you came.**

Overleaf: Devil's Gate Dam in Pasadena.

WEST
SAN GABRIEL
VALLEY

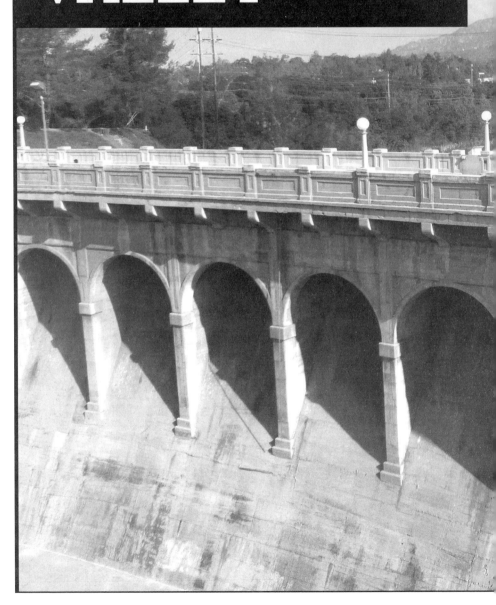

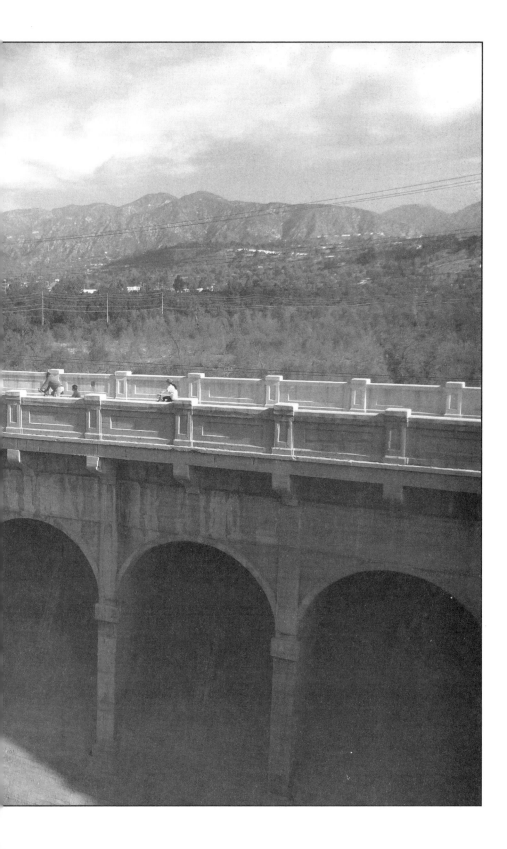

23

GLENDALE

WHISTLING THROUGH A GRAVEYARD

Imagine a magical kingdom of faux European castles, fairy-tale statues, captivating artwork, and a lush, orderly landscape of different "lands." Welcome to Forest Lawn Cemetery—the Disneyland of cemeteries, where even Walt Disney is a permanent visitor.

- ■ **TERRAIN:** Flat with stairs and slight inclines
- ■ **SURFACE:** Paved
- ■ **FIDO FRIENDLY?:** No (not allowed in cemetery)
- ■ **PARKING:** Enter through the gates of Forest Lawn Memorial Park at 1712 Glendale Avenue, Glendale; park in any space on the right side of Cathedral Drive

Pop quiz: What was Southern California's number-one tourist attraction in the mid-1950s, before it was surpassed by Disneyland? Answer: Forest Lawn Glendale. Much as Disney would do decades later with Anaheim orange groves, former general manager Hubert Eaton transformed a dreary 1906 cemetery into a must-see destination that inspires the imagination. He traveled Europe to get ideas for architecture and statues, and commissioned the finest Italian stained-glass artists for his mausoleums. Heck, he even had the trash cans sculpted to look like tree stumps.

Eaton's flamboyancy played well to the Hollywood set—more celebrities are buried here than any place in the world. And yet, despite its kitschy aura, Forest Lawn is vigilant about

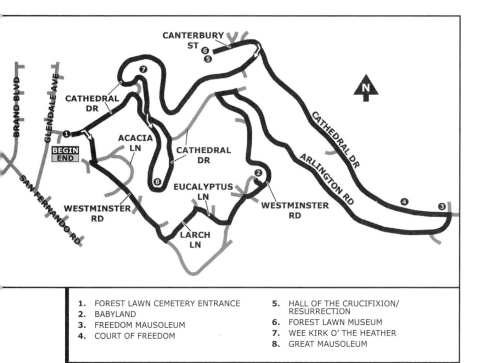

1.	FOREST LAWN CEMETERY ENTRANCE	5.	HALL OF THE CRUCIFIXION/ RESURRECTION
2.	BABYLAND	6.	FOREST LAWN MUSEUM
3.	FREEDOM MAUSOLEUM	7.	WEE KIRK O' THE HEATHER
4.	COURT OF FREEDOM	8.	GREAT MAUSOLEUM

the privacy of its famous internments, refusing to release information about the location of stars' graves. Don't worry, I've done that work for you. As serene as it is unusual, this walk pays tribute to the cemetery's biggest names while navigating its 300 acres of rolling green hills along mostly empty roads.

Park in one of the spaces on Cathedral Drive (feel free to ask the guard at the front gate kiosk for a free map of the grounds). **Walk to the corner, where you'll find a giant sign and a road going east. Turn right at the arrow indicating a church down the street.** Your destination is not the Church of the Flowers, but rather the Wizard of Oz—or, shall we say, the wizard *behind* Oz. Five hundred steps from Cathedral Drive, the headstone of L. Frank Baum is easily visible on the left, where Westminster Road meets Acadia Lane.

Continue walking east on Westminster Road. Behind Baum's grave, up on the bluff, is a Gothic castle. This is the

Great Mausoleum, where Michael Jackson is buried. His body lies in a sarcophagus underneath three stained glass windows. We'll be going inside the mausoleum later to see others' graves, but MJ's is off-limits to the public.

After 400 steps, turn left on Larch Lane. Make a right on Eucalyptus Lane, then a left on Westminster. It quickly takes you to a six-way intersection. Directly in front of you is a statue of an exuberant toddler signifying Babyland—set aside for children five and under.

Continue straight ahead on Westminster. After a few dozen steps, you'll come to a fork. Detour down the left road. After a few paces, you'll encounter a sharp indentation in the curb on the left. It seems randomly placed until you look at an overhead map and realize it forms the point where the bivalves of a heart come together, formed by the roads that cradle Babyland.

Turn around and rejoin Westminster, turning left. The next portion of this walk includes a slow, steady climb

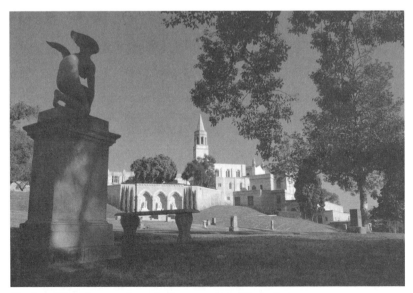

The Great Mausoleum anchors the lower reaches of Forest Lawn.

to the cemetery's upper reaches.

Proceed to the T-intersection with Cathedral Drive and turn right. Continue for about 250 feet, then turn right on Arlington Road. The next 1,600 steps along Arlington are relatively flat and shady, providing the best views of the cemetery and beyond.

> **PICNIC OP**
>
> There are several shaded benches along Forest Lawn's roads that offer nice respites. Use discretion and choose a spot that is a respectful distance from any funeral services.

After curving to the left, Arlington intersects Cathedral Drive again. To your right, on the southeast corner, is a labyrinth carved into the ground. On the northwest corner: the Freedom Mausoleum. **Enter the building from Arlington, through the stained glass doorway that reads "Patriots Terrace."** The first floor contains the tombs of two comic legends—and one forgotten one. The first is Larry Fine, the Chia Pet-haired straight man from the Three Stooges. He's in crypt 22247. Not too far away is Chico Marx (crypt 22018), the Marx Brother with the fake Italian accent. Then there's poor Gummo (21057), the fifth Marx Brother who gave up acting early on and whom almost no one remembers. And you thought it was tough being Zeppo!

Take the flight of stairs near the Arlington entrance up to the second floor. It contains the tombs of Alan Ladd (203582), Clara Bow (203484), Nat King Cole (203692), and George and Gracie Burns (203602), whose epitaph sweetly reads "Together Again."

Find the giant glass doors on the west side of the building and head down the two sets of stairs that face the Court of Freedom. Make a sharp right turn on the concrete walkway, then another right into a little garden behind an unlocked metal gate. Tucked into this cozy corner are the headstones of Walt Disney and three family members. Disney fans regularly honor him by placing trinkets in the hands of a Little Mermaid statue (the mythical version, not the cartoon one). So much for that urban myth about Uncle Walt being stored in a cryogenic freezer . . .

From Disney's land, continue west along the Court of Freedom corridor. Directly north of a thirteen-foot-high George Washington statue are the graves of Errol Flynn and Spencer Tracy in the Garden of Everlasting Peace.

One of the more unique resting spots lies just beyond the soldier at the far end of the Court of Freedom. On the ivied wall of the Immortality section is a tablet with crisscrossed baseball bats honoring Casey Stengel. The Hall-of-Fame manager was, along with Yogi Berra, baseball's poet laureate. One of his colorful quotes serves as his last words on his gravestone: "There comes a time in every man's life, and I've had plenty of them."

To the right of Stengel is the largest mosaic in the world of the signing of the Declaration of Independence, recreated here from John Trumbull's famous painting. One thing that *this* mosaic has that the original doesn't? An endless loop of piped-in Muzak, spilling out of speakers hidden in flower beds. Don't ask me, I just walk here . . .

Return to Cathedral Drive—which is next to Stengel's grave—and continue west. Along the way, you'll pass several statues on the right, including a gargantuan replica of Michelangelo's *David.* Humphrey Bogart, Sammy Davis Jr., and Mary Pickford are buried in gardens near the *David* statue, but their gates are usually locked.

Six hundred steps from the statue, Cathedral makes a sharp left. **Continue going straight onto Canterbury Street,** which ends at a large hilltop parking lot. On the west end of the lot are two buildings. The one on the left is the Hall of the Crucifixion/Resurrection, which contains *The Crucifixion.* At 195 by 45 feet, it's the world's largest religious painting. (If you haven't figured it out yet, bigger is always better here.)

Next stop is the Forest Lawn Museum. Wanna really impress a date? Take him or her up to this free, eclectic museum, which always hosts interesting installations. Over the years, I've seen exhibits covering the art of movie posters, motorcycles, and Marc Chagall—even Lego sculptures have made an appearance. Much like the Hollywood Forever Cemetery's popular movie nights, Forest Lawn's museum redefines what a cemetery can be.

Exit the parking lot by retracing your steps on Canterbury, only this time, when you reach Cathedral, turn right. Follow Cathedral as it languidly winds its way down the lush hillside. At the street's 1,200-step mark is a road sign with an arrow warning cars to "Slow Down." Step off the road to the left and stroll to the black statue of an archer known as "Protection." Six rows to the right of the archer's bow, you'll find the unassuming lawn grave of Jimmy Stewart—befitting of the Everyman actor who played Mr. Smith. Of course, Mr. Stewart also had Scottish ancestry; he rests on a bluff above the Wee Kirk O' the Heather ("Little Chapel of the Lucky Flowers"). **To access the church, continue for several steps down Cathedral Drive, then make a sharp left.**

From the chapel, head 200 steps eastward, past the exit sign. Keep going straight for a few dozen steps to a fork. Both roads, confusingly, are called Cathedral Drive. Take the road on the right, which leads to the Great Mausoleum, the medieval-type castle you saw from below earlier in the walk. Proceed to the mausoleum's entrance. There are several bizarre statues here, including one of a boy riding a goat. It honors Jean Hersholt,

STEPPING BACK

The Wee Kirk O' the Heather is modeled after a fourteenth-century church in Glencairn, Scotland. Built in 1929, it also hosts weddings—another anomaly for a cemetery. Ronald Reagan married his first wife, Jane Wyman, here in 1940.

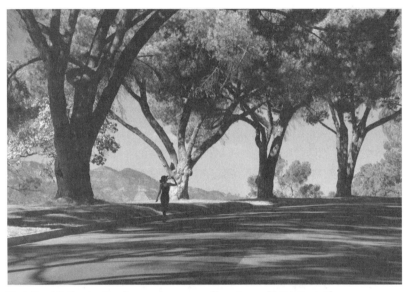

Tree-lined Arlington Road presents commanding views of L.A.'s Eastside.

who wrote and translated Hans Christian Andersen's stories, from which this image is taken.

Step inside the mausoleum. Tell the employee at the front desk that you would like to visit *The Last Supper*, and they'll let you right in. On your way to the replica of that Leonardo da Vinci masterwork, you'll pass several other religious replicas from Michelangelo. At the end of the dimly lit hallway is a large statue of an angel (*In Memoria*). Behind the angel is the crypt of Elizabeth Taylor. Word is, she wanted to be laid to rest near her friend Michael Jackson (who is elsewhere in the building but, again, off-limits to the public). *The Last Supper* is in a separate room to the left, reproduced in stained glass totaling thirty by fifteen feet.

In between the *Last Supper* room and the Elizabeth Taylor angel is a corridor (sometimes chained off) leading to the Sanctuary of Trust, home to the crypts of Carole Lombard and Clark Gable. Lombard was only thirty-three when she died in a plane crash. She was flying back to L.A. to save her marriage to Gable, who reportedly never recovered from his loss and insisted on being buried next to her upon his death eighteen years later. The other corridor worth visiting here

EXTRA STEPS

Looking for a restaurant? There are several bunched around the intersection of Brand Boulevard and San Fernando Road, 600 steps from Forest Lawn's entrance.

is Benediction, which holds the tombs of Jean Harlow, Red Skelton, and impresarios Sid Grauman and Irving Thalberg.

Exit the Great Mausoleum the same way you came in. From there, it's 1,000 steps back to your car. Simply follow Cathedral Drive back to the entrance, making sure you bear left to avoid passing by the Wee Kirk chapel again.

Forest Lawn may not be the Happiest Place on Earth, but for many Hollywood royalty, there clearly is no better place for a final act.

24

UPPER ARROYO SECO

TO HELL AND BACK

Pasadena's Upper Arroyo has a cheery country club feel, but it's not all wine and Rose Bowl. Take this walk to the dark side, where you'll cross over Devil's Gate and pal around with the ghost of England's prince of darkness.

- **TERRAIN:** Flat with stairs, a gradual incline, and one steep, short incline
- **SURFACE:** Mostly unpaved
- **FIDO FRIENDLY?:** Yes
- **PARKING:** Street parking along Rosemont Avenue near the junction of Rose Bowl Drive, Pasadena
- **NOTE:** You may want to avoid this walk on days when there are Rose Bowl events

The Arroyo Seco ("dry stream" in Spanish) is not just a defining feature of Pasadena; it gave birth to the city. In the 1820s, the twenty-five-mile-long seasonal river formed the western boundary of a land grant that would later become Pasadena. It's no coincidence that the wealthiest city-dwellers congregated around the waterway, culminating with the cherry on top in the Rose Bowl. Indeed, the Rose Bowl Loop is one of the more popular walking routes in the Southland. But as you venture farther up the arroyo's Looking Glass, things get curiouser and curiouser.

This walk starts just north of the Rose Bowl. From its intersection with Rose Bowl Drive, head north along Rosemont Avenue, part of the Rose Bowl Loop. Stay on

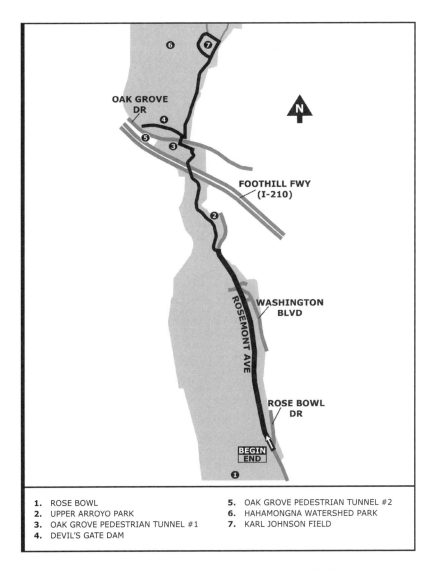

1. ROSE BOWL
2. UPPER ARROYO PARK
3. OAK GROVE PEDESTRIAN TUNNEL #1
4. DEVIL'S GATE DAM
5. OAK GROVE PEDESTRIAN TUNNEL #2
6. HAHAMONGNA WATERSHED PARK
7. KARL JOHNSON FIELD

the left side of the street, where organized chaos prevails between pedestrians and bicyclists making their way around the 3.3-mile perimeter.

If you're looking to fuel up for your five-mile walk, you may want to hit the restaurant at the Brookside Golf Club. Though the golf course is private, the restaurant is open to all and offers superb views of the San Gabriel Mountains and the course itself.

After 1,800 steps, pedestrian traffic peels left down Washington Boulevard as part of the Loop. Your walk, however, **continues straight on Rosemont Avenue. After 400 steps, locate the yellow poles marking a trailhead. Follow this dirt pathway into Upper Arroyo Park,** which hugs the golf course for a few hundred yards before giving way to a riparian wilderness. After passing under the roaring Foothill Freeway (I-210), the trail bends left before reaching a T-intersection with two other trails. **Take the trail to the right,** which quickly leads to a left-leaning buttonhook curve and goes up a steep—but short—grade.

At the top of the trail, you'll reach a fork. To the right is a tunnel. To the left is a concrete stairway leading down the hillside. Take these steps and go straight to Hell. Or so they say. The lore goes back to the Tongva Indians, who believed this mesa was a forbidden place. Flash-forward to Pasadena's first white settlers, who detected the devil himself in rock outcroppings. Things got really bizarro in the 1940s when, under the watchful eye of pagan-worshipper Aleister Crowley, believers of the occult—including a founder of Jet Propulsion Laboratory—started conducting black rituals here, hoping to summon a "moonchild" anti-Christ. Not long thereafter, at least four children disappeared from the area. Legend has it that the black-magic folks succeeded in punching a hole into Hell.

Now, about that stairway . . . gamely follow it to a caged steel ladder and stop there. The ladder drops into the steep walls of the arroyo, leading to a mysterious tunnel dug into the hillside. Portal to Hell, or simply a water control channel? Better to not find out. **Turn around and return to the fork, continuing through the pedestrian tunnel that burrows under Oak Grove Drive.**

On the other side of the tunnel, your vantage point will

change completely. You'll find yourself on the lip of Devil's Gate Reservoir—a giant basin catching storm run-off from the San Gabriel Mountains. When it was built in 1920, the reservoir's

EXTRA STEPS

If you keep walking to the other side of the dam, there's another pedestrian tunnel that goes under Oak Grove. Take that tunnel to get an even better view of the dam's face.

iconic Devil's Gate Dam was an engineering feat whose elegant arches graced postcards. The face of the dam is mostly obscured now by Oak Grove Drive (the street you just walked under), but you can still get a pretty good peek at it.

Head west on the dam's walkway. Note the vintage globe streetlights from the days when cars drove over the levee. As the dam curves slightly, crane your neck over its left wall and look down. Admire the arches, as well as the smooth concrete lines of the dam's 100-foot-tall face.

After your dam detour, walk back to the first tunnel.

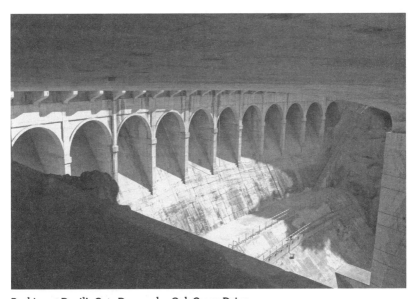

Peeking at Devil's Gate Dam under Oak Grove Drive.

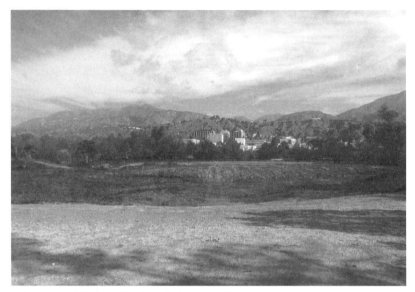

Hahamongna Watershed Park, with JPL in the distance.

Bear left on the wide dirt road that extends into the 300-acre Hahamongna Watershed Park—named after a Tongva chief. The park divides into two parts. The western portion hosts picnic areas and recreational facilities. The eastern edge—where you are—is a network of trails and streams cutting through woodlands and open space, popular with the usual set of dog-walkers, day hikers, and equestrians . . . not to mention resident salamanders and frogs.

After several hundred more steps, you'll arrive at a clearing known as Karl Johnson Field. It doesn't look like much now, but like a lot of things in the L.A. area, its forgotten legacy left behind clues begging to be found. In 1984, city employees, fed up with Pasadena's lack of baseball fields, commandeered this area to create an "unofficial" softball diamond. It didn't last long, as tax-payers cried foul at the idea of maintaining a field that was off-limits to everyone but municipal workers. Remnants of this former Field of Dreams remain. They include a still-functioning water fountain (complete with a "Fido" nozzle), a barbecue, a makeshift snack bar, and even a dilapidated scoreboard, which accounts for the faded billboard-sized placard that otherwise has no purpose being here. There's also a weird silver ball on a slab of concrete bearing the date of the field's dedication.

Karl Johnson Field has since been returned to nature as a water-percolation field. It's also the halfway point of your walk. **Time to return to the ethereal kingdom of Pasadena proper. Simply stay on the trail, which neatly encircles the field in a loop before pointing you in the direction from which you came.**

25

LOWER ARROYO SECO

PHANTOM BIKERS AND PARADISE LOST

Imagine an elevated bicycle superhighway whisking you to downtown L.A. without encountering a single car or pedestrian. On this walk, we'll revisit a time and place when no idea was too bold or too big, and when communing with nature was an American pastime.

- **TERRAIN:** Flat with slight inclines
- **SURFACE:** Paved and unpaved
- **FIDO FRIENDLY?:** Yes
- **PARKING:** Street parking on Arbor Street, near its intersection with Arroyo Boulevard, Pasadena

In the late nineteenth century, as the bourgeoisie were settling in along the Upper Arroyo Seco, bohemians were taking up residence to the south. Not for them were the broad lawns and pretentious palaces of Orange Grove Boulevard. Their ideal abodes were shaded by woodlands and guided by simplicity, with stone foundations and front walls quarried from the arroyo. There is a connectivity to the earth in Pasadena's southern region that you won't find as readily in the north—a connectivity that began over 100 years ago.

Head east on Arbor Street from Arroyo Boulevard. Cross Orange Grove Boulevard and turn left. Half a block later, turn right on the south sidewalk of Del Mar Boulevard. Eighteen hundred steps into your walk—half a block past Fair Oaks Avenue—you'll reach the entrance to Edmondson Alley. Across the street is the nearly 100-year-

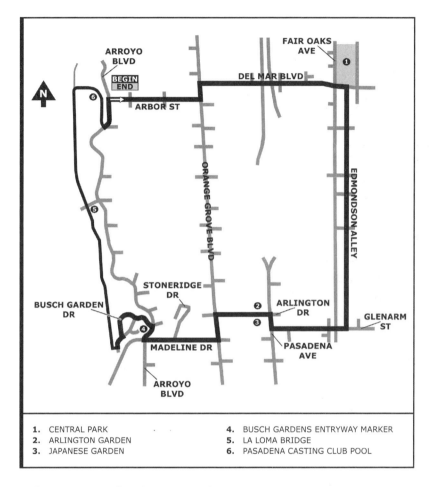

1. CENTRAL PARK
2. ARLINGTON GARDEN
3. JAPANESE GARDEN
4. BUSCH GARDENS ENTRYWAY MARKER
5. LA LOMA BRIDGE
6. PASADENA CASTING CLUB POOL

old Central Park, where sprightly septuagenarians engage in lawn bowling. Meanwhile, on your right, a green street sign points the way down Edmondson Alley. I know your mother always told you never to walk down alleyways, but in this case, she would make an exception because there's history involved.

In the late 1800s, bicycling was all the rage, thanks to mechanical advances that led to the modern bike we know today. Edmondson Alley traces the former route of an elevated wooden bikeway known as the California Cycleway. Its creator, Horace Dobbins, planned an uninterrupted nine-mile path all the way to Olvera Street. The first tollbooth stood right here at the start of Edmondson Alley. Bicyclists paid handsome-

SIDE-STEP

If you choose to abandon the alley at some point, you can always reroute your path to Fair Oaks Avenue, which parallels the alley a half-block west. Rejoin the walk at Glenarm Street.

ly for the privilege—in today's dollars, about $3.00 one-way, $4.50 round-trip. As you **head south on Edmondson,** imagine men with top hats and handlebar mustaches high astride penny-farthings, turning up their noses but not above stealing fleeting glances at the undersides of Victorian-dressed women riding new-fangled two-wheelers.

Your "ride" down Edmondson takes you along the bicycle tollway's first mile before coming to an end at a T-intersection with Glenarm Street. Unfortunately for Mr. Dobbins, his timing was a little off. By the early 1900s, Angelenos were intrigued by a new invention called the automobile. Subsequently, only 1.25 miles of track were laid down. By 1910, the cycleway was dismantled, though its right-of-way did become part of the current Arroyo Seco Parkway (SR 110).

Make a right on Glenarm, staying on the north side. Cross Pasadena Avenue and continue west on Arlington Drive. Just past the corner of Arlington and Pasadena is the entrance to Arlington Garden. Don't let its modest frontage fool you. Entering its portal, you'll find an array of gardens forming a variety of outside "rooms." Other highlights include a wishing tree—on which people hang their wishes—and an actual seven-circuit labyrinth. Every turn of a corner brings a new surprise, with benches and picnic tables sprinkled throughout. The phrase "hidden gem" often gets overused, but it truly does apply to Arlington Garden.

PICNIC OP

Arlington Garden, 275 Arlington Drive.

Leaving Arlington, you may notice a Japanese Garden directly across the street. It's also worth visiting if you happen to catch it on a day it's open to the public, though you may find a sympathetic groundskeeper like I did who will let you mill around anyway.

Continuing west on Arlington Drive, turn left on Orange Grove, then right on Madeline Drive. Enter the ephemeral neverland that made up the original Busch Gardens, as imagined by Adolphus Busch. Unlike the Busch Gardens in Van Nuys that included rides and a monorail that went through a brewery (nothing like imprinting my eight-year-old sensory glands with the smell of fresh beer!), this 1906 version was content with aviaries, waterfalls, and foot-trails through thick foliage to places like the Mystic Hut.

When it closed in 1938, the property was subdivided. But here's the cool part: the neighborhood still bears traces of the old attraction, starting with the mature trees that have soldiered on. On the northwest corner of Madeline and Stoneridge Drive—behind the "Not a Through Street" sign—is a squat stone pillar that once marked the park's boundary. Two blocks away is an even larger monolith. **From Madeline, turn right on Arroyo Boulevard.** The park's original entry marker is at the intersection of Busch Garden Drive and Arroyo. It sat across from the park's admission booth (twenty-five cents for adults; ten cents for kids).

Continue west on Busch Garden Drive. Homes on this street have cleverly cannibalized the park's obsolete structures, their intricate stonework incorporated into front walls and foundations. As you approach the cul-de-sac of Busch Garden Drive, look for a wooden fence to your right. **Find its hidden gate and walk through.** It lets you out onto a dirt trail on the east bank of the Arroyo Seco.

Turn right on the trail, heading north. Pass under the 1914 La Loma Bridge and marvel at its Neoclassical handiwork. At the trail's 2,200-step mark—with the Colorado Street

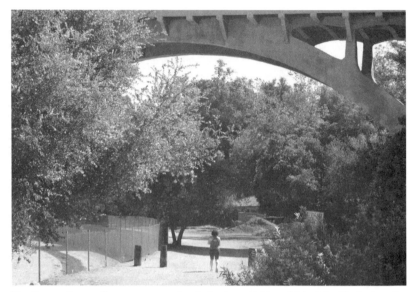

The Arroyo Seco walkway passes under the La Loma Bridge, dubbed the "little sister" of the Colorado Street Bridge.

Bridge forming a majestic backdrop—you'll come to a pedestrian bridge. You are suddenly accosted by people carrying bows and arrows, heading over the arroyo. They're either Roving Archers Club members on their way to an eighty-year-old archery range . . . or reenacting a real-life version of *The Hunger Games*.

Either way, **turn right, away from the pedestrian bridge. Go past the parking lot. As you start to head up the lot's driveway, take a detour to the wide, shallow pool to your right.** While it's tempting to let your dog gallivant through the water, I learned it's best not to, lest you want to subject yourself to stink-eyed glares. Turns out the pool belongs to the Pasadena Casting Club, whose fly-fishing enthusiasts practice their casting here and take things quite seriously.

Head back to the driveway, which lets out at Arroyo Boulevard. Make a left, proceeding one block to Arbor

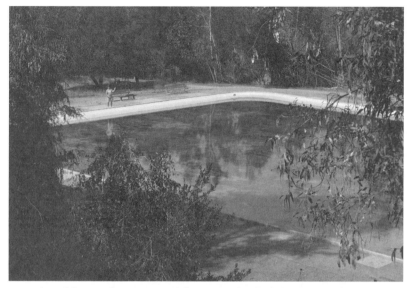

A member of the Pasadena Casting Club practices his fly-fishing techniques.

Street. Just like that, you're back at your point of origin. You started out with the intention of walking through time. But sometimes, you just end up with a wet dog tangled in fishing line.

26

PASADENA

THE ETERNAL CITY BEAUTIFUL

Old never looked so good on a loop that includes Old Pasadena, the Civic Center, and Orange Grove Boulevard—not to mention the site of the second-most-important moonwalk in the history of mankind.

- **TERRAIN:** Flat
- **SURFACE:** Paved
- **FIDO FRIENDLY?:** Yes
- **PARKING:** Street parking on Live Oaks Avenue, just west of its intersection with Orange Grove Boulevard, Pasadena

B y the late 1800s, Pasadena was the premier neighborhood in the Los Angeles area, a West Coast Xanadu for East Coast tycoons looking for balmy winter respites where they could realize their dream mansions. While the newer money tends to gravitate farther west these days, Pasadena's cachet has remained strong, its princely stature and rose-themed traditions unparalleled in Southern California.

From Live Oaks Avenue, follow Orange Grove Boulevard north for one block, then turn left on Arroyo Terrace. Enter the church parking lot driveway to your right (technically Westmoreland Place). At the end of Westmoreland is the Gamble House, a National Historic Landmark considered by many the apex of the American Arts and Crafts movement. It was

ARROYO
TER

GRAND AVE

LIVE OAKS
AVE

HOLLY ST

built in 1908 for David and Mary Gamble of Procter & Gamble fame. Check their website for tours.

Exit the walkway at the end of Westmoreland and turn left on Rosemont Avenue. Make a left on Scott Place, which will take you behind the house. Note the meticulous rock wall on your left—it runs the length of Scott and extends over 1,000 feet! **Turn right on Arroyo Terrace,** gaping at the view of the Rose Bowl and the gorge down below. Next, **hang a left on Grand Avenue,** a shady street with courtly homes of varying architectural styles. **Stay on Grand until you get to Holly Street, the 2,000-step point of the walk. After a quick left, go right on Orange Grove.**

Follow Orange Grove south, across the Ventura

1. GAMBLE HOUSE	**8.** PASADENA CIVIC AUDITORIUM
2. COLORADO STREET BRIDGE	**9.** PASADENA PLAYHOUSE
3. MAXWELL HOUSE	**10.** PASADENA MUSEUM OF CALIFORNIA ART
4. EVERETT HOUSE	**11.** PACIFIC ASIA MUSEUM
5. U.S. COURT OF APPEALS FOR THE NINTH CIRCUIT	**12.** PASADENA CITY HALL
6. TOURNAMENT HOUSE FOR THE ROSE PARADE	**13.** PASADENA PUBLIC LIBRARY
7. NORTON SIMON MUSEUM	**14.** MEMORIAL PARK

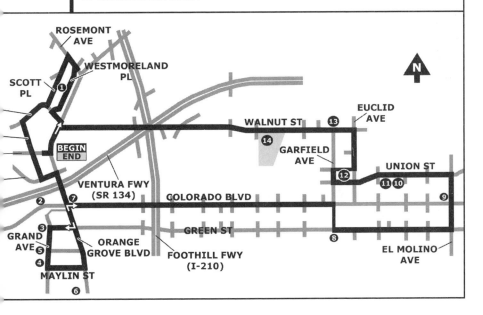

Freeway (SR 134). Turn right on Green Street, which will take you to a T-intersection (Grand Avenue). **Turn left.** The next two blocks, on the west side of the street, showcase several emblematic structures of Pasadena's golden era. Highlights include the 13,000-square-foot Italianate Maxwell House (no relation to the coffee) at 55 Grand, now occupied by a justice foundation, and the Everett House at 171, which used to accommodate the Jet Propulsion Laboratory before giving way to the Shakespeare Club (what was it Hamlet said about "infinite space"?).

EXTRA STEPS

When it was built in 1913, the Colorado Street Bridge was declared the highest concrete span in the world. That designation—combined with the bridge's graceful beauty—made it an irresistible end-point for some, earning it the nickname Suicide Bridge. Walk over this historic landmark by turning right on Grand from Green. At the cul-de-sac, follow the sidewalk to the left for 400 steps as it merges with Colorado.

In the middle of these two buildings is a palatial Mission Revival structure originally built as the Vista del Arroyo Hotel. Its bell tower dominates the east end of the Colorado Street Bridge, as if to say, "Welcome to Pasadena . . . you have *arrived*." After serving high society types in the Roaring '20s, the resort was converted to an Army hospital in the '40s. It's now a branch of the U.S. Court of Appeals for the Ninth Circuit.

From Grand, go east on Maylin Street to Orange Grove. One block south of here, at 391 Orange Grove, is the Tournament House for the Rose Parade, where floats line up every year on January 1st. **Follow Orange Grove north for three blocks to Colorado Boulevard.** On the northeast corner is a 115-foot-tall flagpole dedicated to Pasadeans who served in World War I. Behind the flagpole sits the Norton Simon Museum. Look for *The Thinker* sitting out front, a replica of the original Auguste Rodin statue from the 1880s. While the museum's gallery of paintings are a must-see, less known is its

Sculpture Garden, a maze of free-standing artwork amidst a lake and exotic trees from around the world.

From the Norton Simon, embark on a 2,000-step journey along Colorado through Old Town. Hard to believe it now, but in the 1970s this historic district was in its third decade of urban decline. By the late '80s, its fortunes were on an upswing, creating the thriving hub you see today. Admire the amazing ornamentation of its buildings, most of which date to the 1920s. Find yourself a nice sidewalk café to lunch at and take in the scene.

At 280 Colorado is the massive Paseo Colorado outdoor mall. **Access the walkway that cuts through the courtyard and past the fountain, letting you out on Green Street.** Directly in front of you is the ornate Pasadena Civic Auditorium. Erected in 1931, it's hosted everything from *The Nutcracker* to beauty pageants to the Primetime Emmys. It's also where Michael Jackson first unveiled his signature

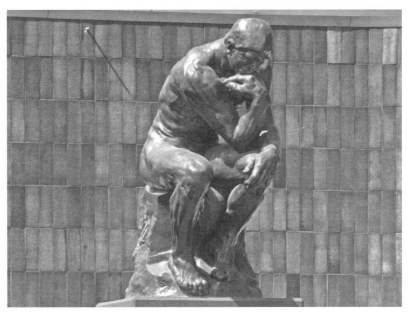

The Thinker reflects on a time without texts and emojis.

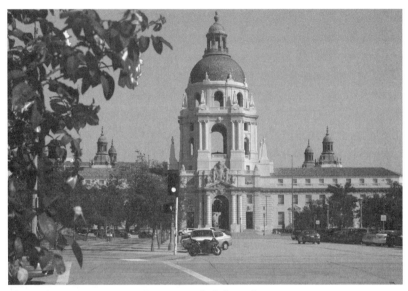

The western entrance to Pasadena City Hall, dedicated in 1927.

"moonwalk" to the American public during a 1983 Motown TV special, simultaneously spawning a generation of Gloved One impersonators on the spot.

Continue east on Green for 800 steps, then turn left on El Molino Avenue. On the west side of the street is the Pasadena Playhouse, a Spanish Colonial Revival venue built in 1925. Tennessee Williams, F. Scott Fitzgerald, and Noel Coward are just some of the playwrights who premiered plays here.

Continue north on El Molino, past Colorado, then go left on Union Street. Pass by the Pasadena Museum of California Art and the Pacific Asia Museum. **When you reach Garfield Avenue, make a right.** As you enter Pasadena's Civic Center, the road turns into a circular plaza like something you'd find in Rome. Not coincidentally, directly to your right is Pasadena City Hall, inspired by the work of a sixteenth-century Italian architect,

PICNIC OP
Memorial Park, 65 Holly Street.

Andrea Palladio. **Stroll through its arched courtyard, exiting at Euclid Avenue.** The city hall is considered a sterling example of the City Beautiful movement, which, inspired by the great European cities, sought to bring aesthetics to urban institutions to promote social harmony. Another Civic Center gem from this era is the Pasadena Public Library at 285 Walnut Street. Locate it by **turning left on Euclid, then left on Walnut.**

Proceed another two blocks on Walnut. On your left is Memorial Park, the west end of the Civic Center district. This is a grand old park with a pavilion for summer performances, with the added bonus of having a Gold Line station right next to it.

From the park, stay on Walnut for another 1,400 steps back to Orange Grove Boulevard. Turn left on Orange Grove and find your car at the intersection of Live Oaks Avenue and a "City Ordinary" World.

27

ALTADENA

PORTAL TO WHITE CITY

Altadena cribs half its name from Pasadena, but this loop reveals a much quirkier place than its posher, more famous neighbor. It also makes its own laws when it comes to gravity. Don't worry, it'll all make sense later.

- **TERRAIN:** Flat with a slight gradual incline
- **SURFACE:** Mostly paved
- **FIDO FRIENDLY?:** Yes
- **PARKING:** Street parking near the intersection of Woodbury Road and Santa Rosa Avenue, border of Pasadena and Altadena

Wedged in an unincorporated section of Los Angeles County along the foothills of the San Gabriel Mountains, Altadena is a portmanteau of the Spanish word "alta" (upper) and "dena" (from Pasadena). The fact that Altadena exists at all is a testament to early, hardy residents who saw their community as having a separate identity from Pasadena, which for years tried to annex it. Still, when it was founded in 1887, Altadena aspired for the same kind of municipal beauty that would come to define its rich neighbor. One of the first things founder John Woodbury did was to plant 134 deodar cedars on both sides of Santa Rosa Avenue, starting at Woodbury Road and leading up to his mansion. **From the Santa Rosa/Woodbury intersection, proceed north on Santa Rosa.** Mr. Woodbury ended up constructing his castle in a different location, but the Himalayan-native cedars did achieve a notoriety of their own.

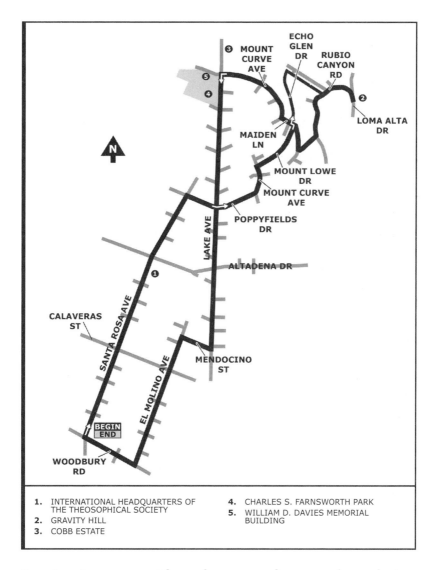

1. INTERNATIONAL HEADQUARTERS OF
   THE THEOSOPHICAL SOCIETY
2. GRAVITY HILL
3. COBB ESTATE

4. CHARLES S. FARNSWORTH PARK
5. WILLIAM D. DAVIES MEMORIAL
   BUILDING

Starting in 1920, residents began to decorate them during the holidays. As noted by signs, the street became known as Christmas Tree Lane, landing it on the National Register of Historic Places. It's worth returning here at night in December to see the "Mile of Christmas Trees" ablaze with 10,000 lights. Of course, even during the day, the majestic trees are

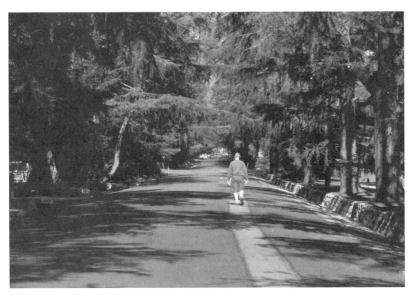

The deodar cedars of Santa Rosa Avenue, aka Christmas Tree Lane.

impressive enough, casting generous shade over the roadway. Notice the weird feature of people's driveways forming little bridges over the street's deep gutters.

Christmas Tree Lane ends at Altadena Drive. The surrounding area is home to many old estates. One of the largest can be spied through a fence to your right. Its grounds form the International Headquarters of the Theosophical Society, promoting a "Oneness of Life" philosophy since 1875.

Proceed another three blocks up Santa Rosa to Poppyfields Drive. Altadena used to have a robust poppy field that was memorialized on postcards like so many long-gone L.A. tourist attractions. In one photo, a Victorian-dressed woman holding a parasol dawdles through a field of orange poppies, with a Craftsman and the San Gabriels framed behind her. The exact location of this former poppy field remains one of Altadena's enduring mysteries. The only clue we have is Poppyfields Drive, which possibly ran alongside it.

Turn right on Poppyfields Drive, cross Lake Avenue,

and stay on Poppyfields until it merges with Mount Curve Avenue. After a block and a half, you'll come to Mount Lowe Drive, which juts off to your right. The street is divided by a grassy median. As you **walk up this street,** look for the historical marker in the grass. As the street name would suggest, it honors a famous railway that used to ferry passengers up nearby Mount Lowe.

The Mount Lowe Railway and Echo Mountain Incline was the brainchild of Professor Thaddeus S. C. Lowe. In the 1890s, he laid down seven miles of steep trolley track to the top of Echo Mountain. Weekend visitors could stay in a Swiss chalet or an eighty-room Victorian hotel, the centerpiece of Lowe's White City, so-called because all the buildings were painted white. Though the resort closed for good in 1936, fossils of it remain. A popular hiking trail mirrors the former "Railway to the Clouds" and ends at Lowe's mountaintop nirvana. Next to the hotel's foundation are the twisted steel gripwheels and cables that pulled the incline up the mountain, bringing home what a massive undertaking Lowe's project was in an era when almost any crazy idea seemed possible . . . and often was.

Mount Lowe Drive ends at Maiden Lane—for vehicles, at least. Since you are not one, **forge ahead through the gate at the T-intersection.** You are now walking on a shaded dirt path known as Echo Glen Drive, a nod to Echo Mountain. **Stay on this trail for 400 steps, until you reach a concrete service road that goes over a culvert.** Do not get on this road! Instead, **access the dirt trail to the right of the road that parallels the culvert. Another 400 steps later, the trail will let you out at Rubio Canyon Road, where you'll make a left.**

Rubio Canyon used to support a pavilion where passengers hopped onto the Great Incline, near the flood control basin to your right. **Stay on Rubio Canyon as it slopes down and circles the basin. Pass over a bridge, at which point Rubio Canyon Road becomes Loma Alta Drive. Follow**

Loma Alta's curvature, passing the driveway of an A-frame house to your left. Make a mental note of this spot. When you complete this walk, return with your car, face it northward (downhill), and slip it into neutral. Look at the horizon out your driver's window as your car begins to roll . . . uphill? What the . . . ?

This stretch of roadway has achieved lore among believers in "gravity hills," inclines that seem to thumb their nose at Sir Isaac Newton. A similar gravity hill exists in the hills above Sylmar. The phenomena are often tied to some purported tragedy, like a school bus that crashed and whose child-spirits are trying to roll your car away from the crash site. So, how to explain *this* optical illusion? Hey, who said it's an optical illusion?

As you ponder Newton's dilemma, **turn around and reconnect with Rubio Canyon Road, taking it to Maiden. Turn right on Maiden, pass Mount Lowe Drive, then turn right on Mount Curve, which intersects Lake**.

Cross over to the other side of Lake. On the southwest corner is Charles S. Farnsworth Park, built by a retired general in the early 1930s. Soak in the impressive stone-built community center, the William D. Davies Memorial Building. It was completed in 1934 by

---

EXTRA STEPS

The Marx Brothers may have been first-rate comedians, but they were lousy landlords. Groucho and company purchased the grand old Cobb Estate in northern Altadena in 1956, but it quickly became dilapidated. Within a few years, marauding teens sacked the unoccupied mansion, leaving behind its foundation and crumpled stairways. Preservationists stepped in, and now the Cobb Estate is a rambling wildlife refuge, its ruins still intact. The grounds can be accessed at the end of Lake Avenue, 300 steps north of its intersection with Mount Curve Avenue.

PICNIC OP

Charles S. Farnsworth Park, 586 Mount Curve Avenue.

Depression-era laborers hired through the Works Progress Administration.

Head south on Lake. Up until 1941, the Pacific Electric Red Car used to run through the middle of Lake, a vital connector to the Mount Lowe Railway. When you reach Calaveras Street, note the picture of a Red Car on the sign for Altadena Plaza. This intersection also hosted the grand opening of the Mount Lowe Railway on July 4, 1893. At its junction with Altadena Drive, Lake morphs into a mom-and-pop district of smoke shops, stationery stores, and dive bars that reflect Altadena's self-effacing character. Drop in for some good eats at a local greasy spoon.

Make a right on Mendocino Street, then turn left on El Molino Avenue. After 1,000 paces, the street intersects Woodbury Road. Turn right on Woodbury, and in two short blocks, you'll be back at your car . . . ready to take on the mystery of Gravity Hill.

Overleaf: Paramount Ranch in Agoura Hills.

SAN FERNANDO VALLEY

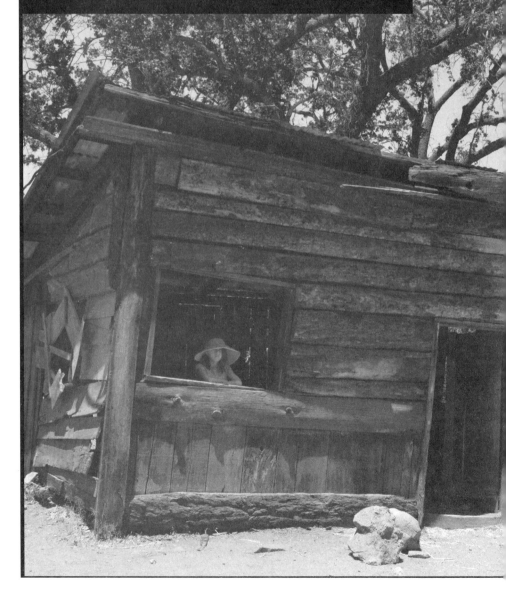

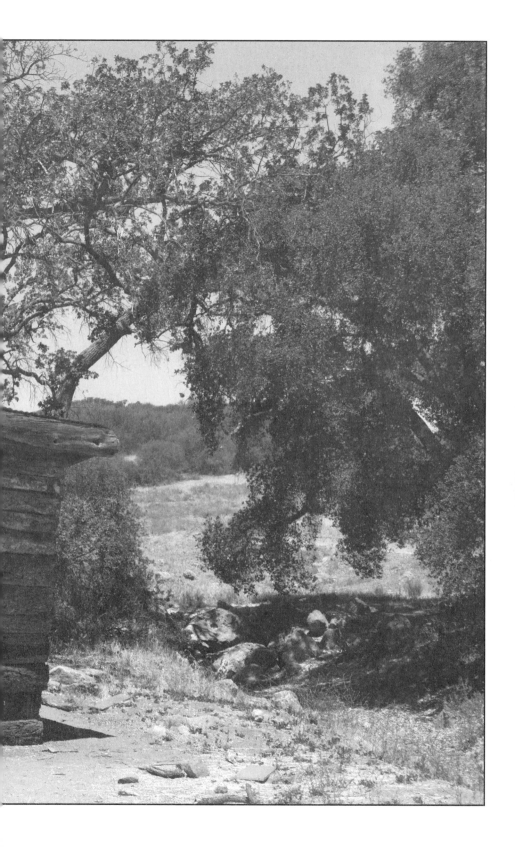

28

AGOURA HILLS

WAY OUT WEST

This out-and-back to Hollywood's hilly backlot includes an intact Western town, the ghost of an old amusement park, and the site where a misguided movie monster learned that humans—unlike flowers—don't float.

- ■ **TERRAIN:** Flat with terraced steps and slight inclines
- ■ **SURFACE:** Paved and unpaved
- ■ **FIDO FRIENDLY?:** Yes
- ■ **PARKING:** Lot for Peter Strauss Ranch at 30000 Mulholland Highway, Agoura Hills

When it comes to shooting movies in the Santa Monica Mountains, Malibu Creek State Park may get "above-the-line" glory, but Peter Strauss Ranch, Lake Malibou, and Paramount Ranch deserve their share of credit.

After parking in the lot for Peter Strauss Ranch, walk toward the lot's entrance. Find the brown sign on the left that reads "Ranch Entrance" and points toward a walking path. Take the path over a bridge paralleling Mulholland Highway and enter the park through a well-marked gate.

To your left is Triunfo Creek. Its once-fertile waters lured Chumash Indians here thousands of years ago. In the 1920s and '30s, developers were equally drawn to it, damming the creek to create Lake Enchanto, an amusement park that included

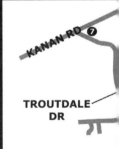

fishing, paddle boats, and a petting zoo. Relics of the park's former glory abound. Conveniently, most of them are just a few hundred steps from the entrance.

Veer to the right and find a collection of structures that includes an aviary and a stone ranch adobe. The house's patio is unique—a terrazzo dance floor with a star. It hosted televised concerts by big bands and top country artists like Johnny Cash.

Just west of the ranch house is a former swimming pool that once accommodated 3,000 people in its 650,000 gallons—largest on the West Coast. It now sits empty behind a fence. Note the bandstand island in the middle of the pool that was used for live performances. (I hope they never plugged in

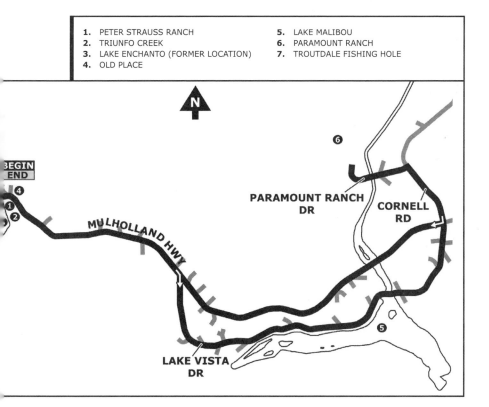

1. PETER STRAUSS RANCH
2. TRIUNFO CREEK
3. LAKE ENCHANTO (FORMER LOCATION)
4. OLD PLACE
5. LAKE MALIBOU
6. PARAMOUNT RANCH
7. TROUTDALE FISHING HOLE

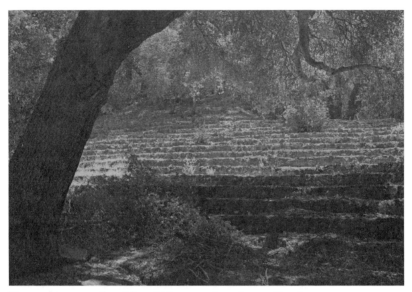

The stone terraces of an old amphitheater at Peter Strauss Ranch.

electrical instruments.)

Southwest of the pool is an old oak with special signifi-cance. It was used as a marker in 1881 in a land grant survey. An upside-down letter "T" was carved in the bark and is still visible today. **From the old oak, climb the terrace of rocks that looks like the side of a Mayan pyramid for a fan-tastic view of the mountains.**

Like so many amusement parks that launched with high expectations, Lake Enchanto could not keep up with the Jone-ses—or the Knotts and Disneys. It closed in the early '60s. Ac-tor Peter Strauss bought the ranch and owned it for a time be-fore donating it to the Santa Monica Mountains Conservancy.

Leaving the ranch, walk back out to Mulholland. Across the street is the Old Place, a rustic bar and restaurant that looks like a weathered hunting lodge. Steve McQueen was known to play poker games in a back room with his celeb-rity friends. A colony of peacocks can often be spotted dart-ing in and out of motorcycles parked out front. If you didn't pack a picnic, this is the only restaurant on this walk, but well worth it for its chili and homemade fruit cobblers alone.

Proceed east on Mulholland, the fifty-five-mile crest line roadway named after water maven William Mulholland. There is very little shoulder here, so be cognizant of traffic. **After 1,800 steps on Mulholland, make a right on Lake Vista Drive** for a pleasant diversion to a little-known lake that abuts the backside of Malibu Creek State Park, where 20th Century Fox shot *M*A*S*H* and the original *Planet of the Apes.*

Lake Malibou (an Anglicized variation of Malibu) is the man-made centerpiece of an exclusive neighborhood that goes back almost 100 years. Though the actual shoreline is off-limits to non-residents, you can still take in the lake's bucolic setting along Lake Vista Drive. Like its counterpart to the south, Lake Malibou hosted dozens of movies and TV shows. Who can forget when Boris Karloff's Frankenstein inadvertently drowns a little girl by chucking her into the water

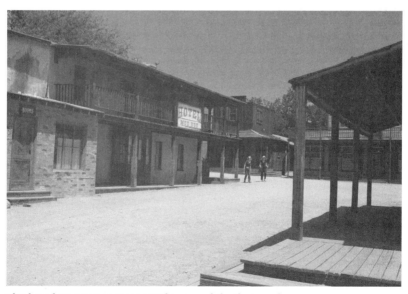

This here faux-Western Town ain't big enough for the two of us.

to see if she floats like a daisy? That famous "oops" scene was shot at the east end of the lake.

PICNIC OP

Paramount Ranch, 2903 Cornell Road. There are tree-shaded picnic tables just south of the Western town.

Once you pass over a bridge, Lake Vista gradually climbs for the next 600 steps. **As it flattens out, continue past Mulholland, where Lake Vista Drive becomes Cornell Road. After another 500 steps, turn left into the "exit" driveway for Paramount Ranch** (technically called Paramount Ranch Drive). You are now at the halfway point—5,000 steps. Before descending into the ranch, take a moment to appraise the lofty mountain with the somewhat pointy peak directly in front of you. If you get a sense of déjà vu, that's because it's believed to have inspired the mountain logo for Paramount Pictures. Its official name is Sugarloaf Peak.

Take the paved road past the parking lot. Step over the bridge that spans a creek. Amble through the park's dusty Western town. Though the ranch was bought by Paramount Pictures in 1927, the studio sold it after World War II to a man named Bill Hertz, who rented it out to production companies under one condition: any structures built for their films must forever remain intact for public enjoyment. Hence the covered wooden sidewalks, sheriff's station, jail, saloon, and old hotel.

EXTRA STEPS

A mere 600 steps from the Peter Strauss parking lot—north on Troutdale to the corner of Kanan Road—is a popular fishing hole that's been around for decades. Troutdale stocks two man-made ponds with rainbow trout. It's where many kids—mine included—hook their first fish. Adults love it, too. A nominal fee gets you a bamboo pole and corn kernels for bait. Find yourself a log bench next to a woodcarved grizzly and cast away. Caught fish cost extra, but who cares when you're taking it home to grill?

There's also a train station left over from *Dr. Quinn, Medicine Woman.*

Like Strauss Ranch, the worthwhile stuff here is conveniently located near the front of the park. While the hiking trails behind the Western town can wait for another day, be sure to explore the creek on your way out of the ranch—it's loaded with crayfish!

Make a right on Cornell to retrace your steps back, with one exception: instead of continuing straight on Lake Vista Drive, turn right on Mulholland Highway, which runs parallel to Lake Vista Drive and will shave off a third of a mile as you sidle back up to your modern covered wagon.

29

CHATSWORTH / SIMI VALLEY

ROCKETS, SHOOT-OUTS, AND BURNOUTS

This walk traverses the border between the counties of Los Angeles and Ventura, a mysterious region where the present is always bumping up against the past—road and rail, stucco and stone, Hope and Crash, and crooning cowboy and singing serial killer.

- ■ **TERRAIN:** Flat with slight inclines
- ■ **SURFACE:** Paved and unpaved
- ■ **FIDO FRIENDLY?:** Yes
- ■ **PARKING:** Lot for Corriganville Park, 7001 Smith Road, Simi Valley

The northwest San Fernando Valley is L.A.'s own badlands—a foreboding outcrop of sandstone caves and gravity-defying boulders perched on mountaintops. No wonder it's drawn so many sects and communes over the years. Before the infamous Manson Family took up residence here in the 1960s, it saw the likes of the Pisgah Grande, the Great Eleven Club, and the WKFL Fountain of the World, which endured its own bloodbath in 1958.

And yet it's not just a coincidence that Charles Manson's brood took over an old Western movie set. For decades, Hollywood studios were similarly drawn to the dramatic landscape. This mixed legacy of the occult and popular entertainment has given the boundary between Chatsworth and Simi Valley a strange duality. For this walk, we'll keep our feet firmly planted in the lightness.

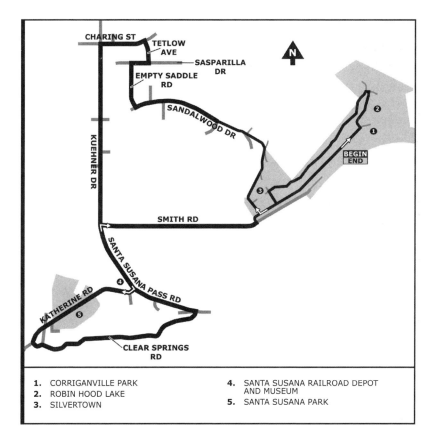

1. CORRIGANVILLE PARK
2. ROBIN HOOD LAKE
3. SILVERTOWN

4. SANTA SUSANA RAILROAD DEPOT AND MUSEUM
5. SANTA SUSANA PARK

From the dirt parking lot of Corriganville Park, walk toward the sign at the east end of the lot to access an interpretive trail. The park is named after a former movie stuntman named Ray "Crash" Corrigan. When it opened in 1949, families came from all over the Southland for the stunt shows, shoot-outs, and stagecoach rides set against a Western town known as Silvertown. By the late '50s, Corriganville Park was so popular, it was drawing larger crowds than Disneyland several years after the Magic Kingdom opened for business.

The best way to see Corriganville is to simply wander its trail loop, which includes twenty markers outlining the history of the 206-acre site. The most interesting remnant of the park is its now-empty watering hole, Robin Hood Lake, which was featured in dozens of Westerns. Don't miss the concrete bunker with portholes at its west

> **PICNIC OP**
>
> Lakeside at Corriganville Park, 7001 Smith Road.

end—it was used to shoot underwater scenes from the Johnny "Tarzan" Weissmuller movie *Jungle Jim.* On the northern shore is a faux-rock ledge extending over the basin. Known as Stunt Rock, it's where many a villain or hero were shot off the crag and plunged into the water. Gene Autry (or at least a good double) can be seen tumbling off of it in the movie poster for *Hills of Utah.* The former lake is surrounded by shaded benches and boulders—ideal vantage points from which to imagine all the shoot-'em-up action that once unfurled in the lake before you.

While the old sets are fun to navigate, nature puts on a pretty cool show here as well. Secret caves, a trickling stream, and a forest of centuries-old oak trees remind you why Crash fell for this place to begin with. As you **loop back to the parking lot on the northern trail,** check out the gnarled old oak trunk that somehow muscled its way through a big rock.

Just north of the parking lot are the concrete foundations of an old barn. After Bob Hope bought the ranch in 1965—renaming it Hopetown—most of the structures burned down. This spot includes the former main drag of Silvertown, which sat in for Tombstone and Dodge City in movie Westerns. You should have logged about 1,000 steps by this point.

Continue past the parking lot, toward the entrance where you drove in. Right before the dirt road bears left between a row of eucalyptus trees, find another dirt road to your right. **Take this trail, which is identified on maps as Sandalwood Drive.** (If you find yourself back on the pavement of Smith Road, you've gone a few feet too far.) After skirting behind Silvertown, the trail climbs a slope and bends left.

Six hundred steps later, Sandalwood exits an open gate and turns into blacktop, plopping you into the type of cook-

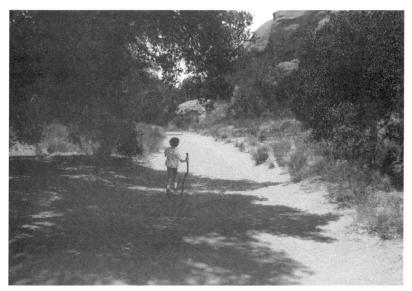

Nature has reclaimed Crash Corrigan's once-thriving Western empire.

ie-cutter 1980s neighborhood you'd find in the movie *E.T.* Welcome to Hopetown Estates—219 stucco-heavy homes cleaved out of the ranch's former lower section. As you **trot down Sandalwood,** you'll find street names that are all that remain of the former Western town: Cowboy Street, Cody Avenue, and, my favorite, Chaps Court.

From Sandalwood, turn right on Empty Saddle Road, right on Sasparilla Drive, then left on Tetlow Avenue. (Tetlow does not allow vehicle access at its mid-point, but the sidewalks continue unabated.) **Make a left on Charing Street and another left on Kuehner Drive, leaving Hopetown behind. Stay on the east side of Kuehner.** Follow the curvy sidewalk for 1,200 steps until you get to an A-framed restaurant with a covered wagon out front called the Old Susana Café. Inside are old photos of Corriganville and former stagecoach routes. This is a must-stop for one of their delicious comfort-food meals. If you brought your dog, find a seat on the pet-friendly patio with lots of shade.

Exiting the restaurant, continue another 800 steps on Kuehner. Pass the first Katherine Road on your right, then pass over the bridge that spans the railroad tracks. Just past the tracks, turn right on the second Katherine Road (the correct one!). On your right, you'll see a two-story yellow building with brown trim—the Santa Susana Railroad Depot and Museum. The station was built in 1903. If it's a weekend afternoon, step inside the museum. It includes a recreation of the depot's waiting room and is staffed by friendly old-timers who will show you how to send a telegram ("More reliable than a cell phone," I was told, and I couldn't disagree). Next to the museum are coveralled train hobbyists perpetually fiddling with a massive train set that includes a scale replica of the entire Los Angeles area. There's also a model of Corriganville's golden age. Don't forget to grab some freshly popped popcorn on your way out!

Leaving the depot's parking lot, proceed west on Katherine. As you pass by scenic Santa Susana Park, you'll see another jarring transition in the landscape. The road narrows and the homes get all funky-looking with rambling yards. Hopetown Estates, this ain't—it looks more like Topanga Canyon. In actuality, you're now in an unincorporated slice of Simi Valley known as Santa Susana Knolls. Nestled at the base of the Santa Susana Mountains, the Knolls used to house many of the 6,000 employees from Rocketdyne, where rocket engines were built and tested. During the height of the Cold War Era, residents regularly heard thunderous booms that rattled windows, with mysterious smoky lights illuminating the nighttime sky.

About a block past Santa Susana Park, turn left on Clear Springs Road. This even narrower lane is heavily shaded and lined with shotgun shacks that were primarily designed as hunting cabins or weekend retreats. A Santa Susana Hills prospectus from the 1920s promised city-dwellers a utopia with "no poisonous insects," clear mountain spring water, and steep peaks that "will tax the stamina of the most experienced nimrod."

Stay on Clear Springs Road for 1,000 steps, then turn left on Santa Susana Pass Road. Note the rundown strip mall on the corner. (The Santa Susana Train Depot features several historical photos of this site.) In its heyday, the center included a biker bar where Arnold Schwarzenegger filmed scenes from *The Terminator* in the parking lot. Visitors over the tavern's seventy-three years included everyone from screen hero John Wayne to failed rocker Charlie Manson, whose Spahn Ranch hideaway was just two miles east of here, off Santa Susana Pass Road. What was that we said about the area's duality?

From here, it's about 1,000 steps back to your car. **Simply continue on Santa Susana Pass Road until it turns into Kuehner, then turn right on Smith Road.**

EXTRA STEPS

If you want to experience more of the rustic beauty of Santa Susana Knolls, the neighborhood continues for about another mile to the west. Simply continue on Katherine Road.

30

SEPULVEDA DAM

THE VALLEY'S PHILHARMONIC

What do you get when you cross two lakes, three creeks, and a 2,000-acre park? Sepulveda Wildlife Reserve, a little piece of paradise just north of Sepulveda Dam that pleases the ears as much as the eyes.

- **TERRAIN:** Flat
- **SURFACE:** Paved and unpaved
- **FIDO FRIENDLY?:** No (not allowed in Sepulveda Wildlife area)
- **PARKING:** Lot for Woodley Park at 6350 Woodley Avenue, Van Nuys; park as far east as you can, past the cricket fields, in the lot next to the west shoulder of the San Diego Freeway (I-405)

You're stuck in gridlock near the 405 and 101 Freeway interchange—their default state. Bored, your eyes drift off through the windshield. They land on that familiar landmark in the corner of the Valley where Encino and Van Nuys come together: the Sepulveda Dam, a streamlined concrete fortress . . . doing *what*, exactly? It doesn't look like a dam in the traditional sense. That's because it was designed to merely regulate water flow, not hold it back, much like the Valley's other dams and channels that went up after the 1938 flood that killed over 100 Angelenos.

The happy upshot of the Sepulveda Dam's existence? A massive recreational area in its flood control basin, providing much-needed green space for both people and wildlife

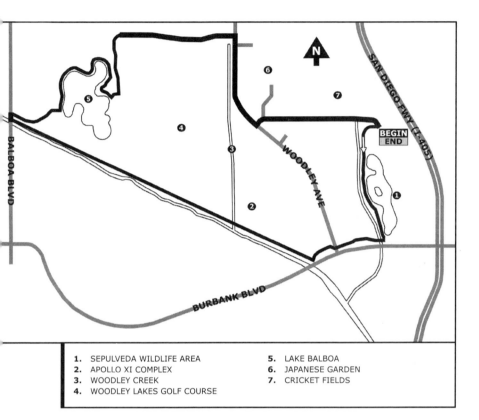

1. SEPULVEDA WILDLIFE AREA
2. APOLLO XI COMPLEX
3. WOODLEY CREEK
4. WOODLEY LAKES GOLF COURSE
5. LAKE BALBOA
6. JAPANESE GARDEN
7. CRICKET FIELDS

in the region.

From the parking lot near the 405 Freeway, follow the foot trail at the lot's southwest corner that leads toward the restrooms. A stone sign greets you: "Sepulveda Wildlife Area: A Symphony of Sounds." It starts with the constant hum of the freeway. Annoying traffic? Nah, think of it as white noise, akin to the gentle rippling of ocean waves!

Within minutes, you are in another world. The concrete pathway turns to dirt, grass gives way to flora, and a creek appears on your right. Four hundred steps in, a lake enters the picture on your left, fed by recycled water from the Tillman Water Reclamation Plant. Mellifluous bird sounds take over, a harmonic convergence of chirps, trills, and whistles, with duck and geese honks providing baritone notes. This is arguably the best place to bird-watch in the Valley, and bird-watchers know it, regularly turning out here with binoculars in tow. Signs help identify the differences between cormorants, herons, and egrets. In the winter, you'll see flocks of Canada geese; in the spring, ducklings with their mamas. Birds aside, this is also just a peaceful spot to hang out in for a while.

At the 1,000-step mark, swing right on a trail that goes over the creek. It makes a sharp left and curves southward toward the intersection of Woodley Avenue and Burbank Boulevard. Cross Woodley at this intersection and pick up the paved walkway/bikeway on the northwest corner. Just before the walkway goes over the bridge of the Los Angeles River, turn right on the dirt path that parallels the river's northern bank. This stretch of waterway is refreshingly untamed, its willows and sandy bottom affording more wildlife opportunities. Like the Glendale Narrows farther south, it's open to non-motorized boaters during the summer.

As you loaf along the river, you may hear a loud buzzing that sounds like ginormous mosquitoes. In a field on your right, just before Woodley Creek, model airplanes and helicopters often swoop through the sky. They're controlled by members of the Valley Flyers, who have been barnstorming their aircraft here for over sixty-five years. The group's Apollo XI complex includes runways and helicopter pads. If you like air shows, come back in December, when the Flyers host a mini-me version of one.

Continue past the Woodley Lakes Golf Course. After logging 2,800 steps along the river, hang a right on Balboa Boulevard, then another right on the pathway that takes you to Lake Balboa and Anthony C. Beilenson Park. Head to the shoreline to access a hiking trail that circumnavigates the manmade lake, then simply make either a right or a left until you get to Lake Balboa's eastern shore. Unlike the first lake, this one allows fishing and is geared toward recreation.

From the lake's eastern edge, head a few paces east to a park road (watching for vehicular traffic) and turn left. The road curves to the right, hugging the northern boundary of the golf course, and lets out at Woodley Avenue. Again, watching for cars, cross the street and make a right on Woodley.

PICNIC OP

Lake Balboa, 6300 Balboa Boulevard. Anywhere along the grassy shoreline.

EXTRA STEPS

As the parking lot sign indicates, Sepulveda Basin has a Japanese Garden. After turning into the driveway that returns you to your car, bear left at the fork to get to it. The immaculate grounds include a lakeside tea room and origami demonstrations, its waters replenished by the Tillman Reclamation plant next door. Check their website to make sure they'll be open—they're typically closed Fridays and Saturdays.

As Woodley veers away from the golf course, you may hear the familiar buzzing of the model airplanes. You are now on the other side of the Apollo XI field. This is also your cue to **head left into the parking lot where you began your walk (the first driveway will take you there—look for the signs for the Cricket Fields and a Japanese Garden).** It's 500 steps to your car. Time to leave the Symphony of Sounds and return to the cacophony of the city.

31

VALLEY GLEN

HOW GREEN IS OUR VALLEY!

Oddly, there is no glen in Valley Glen, but you will find a two-and-a-half-mile greenbelt, an unlikely stream, and a Great Wall that may not rival China's, but is worth seeing just the same. Just don't visit the wall when it rains lest it disappear before your eyes.

- **TERRAIN:** Flat
- **SURFACE:** Paved and unpaved
- **FIDO FRIENDLY?:** Yes
- **PARKING:** Street parking near the intersection of Coldwater Canyon Avenue and Chandler Boulevard, Valley Glen

It's easy to dismiss the central San Fernando Valley as an unredeemable patchwork of tacky strip malls, parking lots, and psychics. If that's all you see, then this walk is the perfect antidote for those prejudices.

From Chandler Boulevard, head north on Coldwater Canyon Avenue, keeping to the east side of the street. Here you'll find the Tujunga Greenbelt, a shaded, grassy pathway that overlooks the Tujunga Flood Control Channel, which feeds the Los Angeles River downstream. After 400 steps, the wash goes under Burbank Boulevard. **Jump over to the left side of Coldwater Canyon, where the greenbelt continues alongside the channel.** This is where the good stuff starts.

Look down at the western wall of the wash and note the start of a half-mile-long mural. The Great Wall of Los Angeles

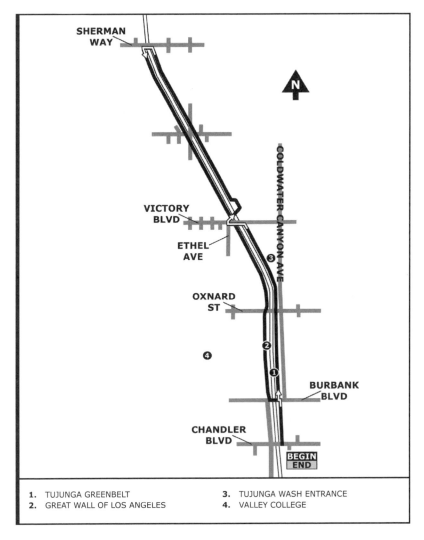

1. TUJUNGA GREENBELT
2. GREAT WALL OF LOS ANGELES
3. TUJUNGA WASH ENTRANCE
4. VALLEY COLLEGE

displays a pictorial history of California from the dinosaur days to the modern era. What makes this mural so special—besides the fact that it's the longest in the world—is that it was painted mostly by 400 young adults under the supervision of artist Judith F. Baca. Starting in 1974 and continuing well into the '80s, Baca and her team added different epochs every summer. My grandmother used to live just north of this mural. Whenever we drove by over the years, I marveled at how long it was getting and wondered, "Will it ever end?" Maybe not. Baca's goal is to keep adding newer decades to California's history and reach the one-mile mark.

A little past Oxnard Street, the greenbelt/wash swings left of Coldwater Canyon. **Go through the pedestrian gate, step onto the decomposed granite trail,** and enter the Tujunga Wash Ecosystem Restoration Project, the beginning of a 3,000-step march toward Sherman Way. While you won't exactly forget your urban surroundings, it's always surprising how transformative the experience of walking along a nature trail can be. Willows, alders, and cottonwoods line the walkway, along with more than a dozen species of perennial shrubs and native grasses. This is a beautifully realized park, dotted with benches and plenty of kiosks documenting the history of this area of the Valley.

When you get to Victory Boulevard, the Tujunga Wash trail ends abruptly before picking up again just north of the thoroughfare. To re-access it, **turn left on Victory and go half a block to Ethel Avenue. Make a right on Ethel, crossing the Tujunga Wash bridge.** In front of you is a sea of hot asphalt, the parking lot for a soulless shopping center. This is exactly the type of Valley monstrosity you were trying to escape! Unfazed, you lower your head, **power fifty steps northwest of the lot, and find the re-access point for Tujunga Wash** as you feel your blood pressure returning to normal.

EXTRA STEPS

Just east of Coldwater Canyon, Chandler enters a micro-neighborhood that is home to the largest concentration of observant Jews in the Valley—many tracing their roots to Israeli, Russian, and Iranian immigrants from the 1980s. Businesses along the Chandler corridor are an eclectic mix of kosher butchers, shops, and synagogues, with most families living in the ranch houses just north of the boulevard.

Continue on the greenbelt for 2,200 steps, at which point you'll reach Sherman Way. Exit through the gate and make a left on the sidewalk. Walk a few paces over the bridge and re-enter the park on the west bank of the wash (can washes have banks?). You've just about hit the halfway point and are now ready to head back.

With its native plants

> **STEPPING BACK**
>
> Northeast of Burbank and Coldwater Canyon are three transmission towers rising up about a quarter-mile away. They were built in the 1940s by Loyd Sigmon, the director of engineering for KMPC Radio. Sigmon's place in history would be immortalized in 1955, when he invented the Sig Alert, a phrase known all too well by every Southland driver encountering traffic jams. Now, if someone could just find a way to get rid of traffic jams, I guarantee that their name would trump Loyd Sigmon's.

and dirt walkway, this side of the wash is similar to the other, but it has an added bonus: a stream. Or, as the signs say, a "meandering stream," meant to hark back to the original Tujunga waterway before it was paved over in the early 1950s. The stream parallels the trail for much of its length before disappearing into the wash through a system of settling ponds, pipelines, and riparian vegetation absorption. Interpretive signs do a far better job of explaining how the whole thing works than I could ever do here.

Continue on the west bank past Oxnard, where it abuts Valley College. You are back to the stretch of wash that hosts the mural, although you can't see it from this side. **When you reach Burbank Boulevard, cross over to the southeast corner of Burbank and Coldwater Canyon.**

It's just a few short steps to your departure point at Coldwater Canyon and Chandler, and yet a long way from the clichés of the Valley whence we all came.

32

STUDIO CITY

SHADES OF MAYFIELD

Whether it's an old-timey golf course, a kitschy hotel, or a burger joint set in a vintage train, this Studio City loop showcases the Valley the way we like it—a modern suburbia that hasn't forsaken its past.

- **TERRAIN:** Flat
- **SURFACE:** Paved and unpaved
- **FIDO FRIENDLY?:** Yes
- **PARKING:** Street parking near the intersection of Coldwater Canyon Avenue and Moorpark Street, next to the Little Brown Church in the Valley at 4418 Coldwater Canyon Avenue, Studio City

In 1952, a B-movie actor named Ronald Reagan married Nancy Davis in the Little Brown Church. With its dollhouse-like low ceiling, the cathedral looks like the perfect place of worship for cinematic Munchkins—appropriate, perhaps, since it opened the same year as *The Wizard of Oz*. Since then, its doors have quite literally remained open 24/7; you can drive by at 2 AM and look directly into the chapel.

This small treasure at the intersection of Coldwater Canyon Avenue and Moorpark Street is the starting point for a walk through Studio City, where "comfort" landmarks with the coziness of a presidential fireside chat still abound.

From the church, proceed 1,000 steps east on Moorpark. Turn right on Whitsett Avenue. After two blocks, you'll come to the Weddington Golf and Tennis complex on your right. Duck inside its unfussy clubhouse, whose faintly

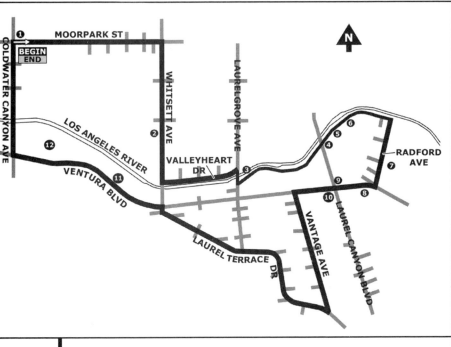

1. LITTLE BROWN CHURCH IN THE VALLEY
2. WEDDINGTON GOLF AND TENNIS COMPLEX
3. LOS ANGELES RIVER GREENWAY PARK
4. GREAT TOAD GATE
5. BUTTERFLY GARDEN
6. RATTLESNAKE WALL
7. CBS STUDIO CENTER
8. DU-PAR'S RESTAURANT & BAKERY
9. *FROM PROSPECTOR TO DIRECTOR* MURAL
10. FOX STUDIO CITY THEATRE (FORMER LOCATION)
11. CARNEYS
12. SPORTSMEN'S LODGE

musty odor betrays six decades of cigarette smoke, golfer sweat, and steamy Valley summers. Swill a milkshake in its small café. Out back, the golfing faithful take whacks on the driving range and queue up for the par 3 nine-hole.

Continue south on Whitsett. Turn left on Valleyheart Drive, a shady residential street that hugs the Los Angeles River. **Four blocks later, you'll reach an intersection with Laurelgrove Avenue. Pivot to your right and find the footbridge that crosses over the river. On the other side of the bridge, take the ramp down to a pathway that runs alongside the south bank.** You've entered the Los

Angeles River Greenway
Park, a wending trail with
native landscaping that
continues for the next
1,200 steps. Keep an eye

out for piles of rocks fused together to look like chairs. These
are actual seating areas where you can take a load off, proving
that the best kind of art is that which you can sit on.

Farther downriver, head up the ramp to Laurel Canyon Boulevard. Cross the street at the crosswalk and descend the ramp on the other side. The greenway continues through the Great Toad Gate, which was designed by a student at a nearby school. The highlights of this section are a Butterfly Garden and Rattlesnake Wall, which is topped by a massive stone rattlesnake with intricately carved scales and a menacing face. The serpent's slithering body disappears underground, only to have its tail re-emerge unexpectedly out of the earth a few feet later. A similar snake appears at Rattlesnake Park several miles down the river—perhaps its cousin?

The greenway ends a few steps later. **Go up the concrete ramp and turn right on Radford Avenue. Cross over to the east side of the street.** On your left you'll find a historic production lot built in 1928 by silent movie producer Mack Sennett—the inspiration for the name Studio City. Now known as the CBS Studio Center, it's where cultural touchstones like *Leave It To Beaver*, *The Mary Tyler Moore Show*, and *Seinfeld* were filmed. Plaques on Radford's sidewalk memorialize famous productions that were shot here (wait . . . Jennifer Lopez's *Enough* gets a plaque? Really?). The lagoon from *Gilligan's Island* used to reside on this lot, too, but was paved over for a parking lot. The SS *Minnow* is truly lost now.

Reaching Ventura Boulevard, make a right. Pie lovers, rejoice: across the street is Du-Par's Restaurant & Bakery, a Valley staple that is one of the few remaining places in L.A. where you can still get an all-rhubarb pie. As you continue

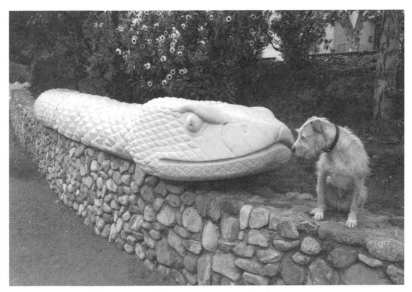

That's odd . . . it looks like a rattlesnake, but it doesn't smell like one.

westward, you'll come to a bank on the northeast corner of Ventura and Laurel Canyon that used to be a Home Savings and Loan. Admire the 1970 mural, *From Prospector to Director*, which charts the history of L.A. in four different vignettes. It was designed by Millard Sheets, one of dozens that the famous painter created across the Southland in the mid-twentieth century.

Cross over to the southwest corner of Laurel Canyon and Ventura. At this point, Ventura enters a vibrant business district. As you **continue west,** you'll encounter the former Fox Studio City Theatre at 12136 Ventura, just a few steps from the corner. It's now a bookstore, but vestiges remain, like the terrazzo floor, neon marquee, and stand-alone box office.

Briefly ditching the boulevard's hustle and bustle, **hang a left on Vantage Avenue. Proceed a half-dozen blocks to Laurel Terrace Drive and turn right.** Laurel Terrace is a shady stroll past handsome clapboard homes with picket fences. **Follow Laurel Terrace until it merges into Whitsett**

at Ventura. Turn left onto Ventura's northern sidewalk.

About this time, you will have worked up an appetite, and a good thing, too. Your next stop

SIDE-STEP
If you're looking to shave some steps off—and window-shopping is more your thing—simply stay on Ventura Boulevard. Rejoin the main route at Whitsett.

is Carneys at 12601 Ventura—a Studio City hot dog and hamburger joint housed in an old yellow Union Pacific passenger train. (The original Carneys is on the Sunset Strip.) Pink's Hot Dogs may get all the hype, but for my money, if there's a more mouthwatering dish than Carneys' split-and-grilled sauerkraut hot dog with chili peppers and grilled onions, this mouth has yet to find it.

From Carneys, continue west on Ventura. In 600 steps, you'll encounter the granddaddiest of all Studio City landmarks, known as the Sportsmen's Lodge. How old is this rustic-themed resort? Just as Beverly Hills coalesced around the

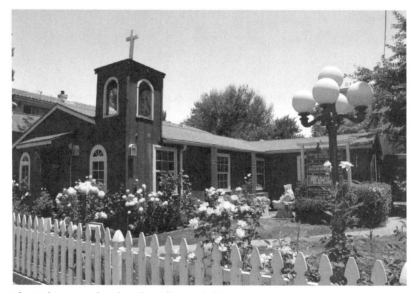

The Little Brown Church in the Valley is a holdover from the FDR era.

Beverly Hills Hotel, Studio City grew up around Sportsmen's Lodge. It began as a trout-filled fishing hole in the 1880s. Then, during Hollywood's Golden Age, its lounge emerged as a celebrity sanctuary. Channel that fancy-free era as you lope along the lodge's foot-bridges. Imagine Bette Davis throwing back martinis through the bar's window while John Wayne teaches his kids how to fish in its ponds. Or maybe you're just here to crash a wedding reception in its banquet hall, like the one Ronald and Nancy Reagan held after getting married at the Little Brown Church.

Ah, yes, the place where it all began. The Gipper obviously had a soft spot for Studio City. As you return to the church—**500 easy steps north on Coldwater Canyon**—so now do you.

33

NORTH HOLLYWOOD

NOHO'S FREEWAY TO NOWHERE

No one will ever mistake Whitnall Highway for a scenic parkway. But underneath its strands of power lines lies the graveyard of a proposed freeway that makes for a unique Valley walk rife with unexpected treasures.

- **TERRAIN:** Flat
- **SURFACE:** Mostly paved
- **FIDO FRIENDLY?:** Yes
- **PARKING:** Street parking near the intersection of Whitnall Highway and Cleon Avenue, North Hollywood

You find yourself in Hollywood, living in an apartment on N. Bronson Avenue. A buddy in Northridge is hosting an impromptu Friday night dinner party. Can you make it?

You do the math in your head. Three freeways in rush-hour traffic: the 101, the 405—maybe even the 118. It'll take you ninety minutes to get there. Then you remember there's a freeway that burrows under the Hollywood Sign and spits you out at Forest Lawn, where it then cuts diagonally across the Valley like a wormhole through time and space. You tell your friend you'll be there in thirty minutes. You make it in twenty.

Sure, it sounds likes fantasy. But as recently as the 1960s, the Whitnall Freeway still appeared on proposed freeway maps. City planners eventually came to their senses about blasting an eight-lane, two-mile tunnel through the heart of the Santa Monica Mountains. Still, grading had already

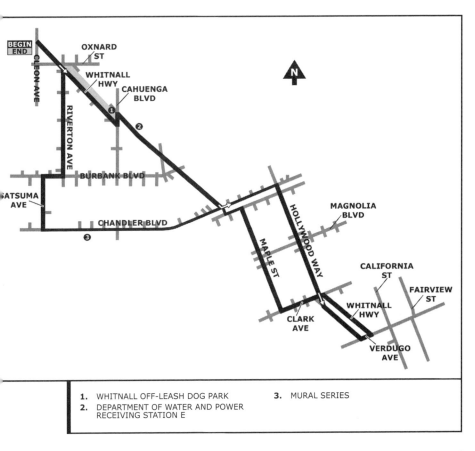

1. WHITNALL OFF-LEASH DOG PARK
2. DEPARTMENT OF WATER AND POWER RECEIVING STATION E
3. MURAL SERIES

started for the freeway-that-never-was in a section north of Burbank, just past Oxnard Street. For proof, you're going to walk it yourself.

Start on the sidewalk at the intersection of Cleon Avenue and Whitnall Highway (as it's now called), and head southeast. Notice how Whitnall—named after city planner George Whitnall—is indeed the width of a freeway, with opposing lanes separated by a wide median. This right-of-way is now dominated by high-voltage electrical wires, buzzing and stretching as far as the eye can see toward Mount Lee in the distance (the very same mountain that the freeway would've plowed through).

The first block passes a depressed business district that has seen better days. In the 1970s and early '80s, one of the storefronts had the words "Jhon's Shoe Repair" glued to the window. It belonged to my grandfather, John. The signmakers misspelled his name and he never bothered to change it. Next to his shop was a Goodwill drop-off bin that bored teenagers used to light on fire. On second thought, maybe there were no "better days" here. Don't worry, things will get better . . .

Continue down the sidewalk for two more blocks. On your left, the dirt median gives way to the Whitnall Off-Leash Dog Park, one of the bigger ones in the city. If you brought your dog, here's your chance to let it loose as you ponder the definition of "progress." In this case, score one for the local community, brought together by this park instead of divided by convoys of big rigs.

Just past the dog park is Cahuenga Boulevard. **Cross Cahuenga, turn left, and then turn right on Whitnall Highway North.** On your left you'll find one of those classic Art Deco Department of Water and Power buildings—"Receiving Station E." Oddly, this one seems to have a Mayan frieze. Or is it Polynesian? Forget it, Jake, it's Whitnall Highway.

Keep walking until you reach Chandler Boulevard. You've now logged about 2,400 steps. Though the power lines still run overhead, Whitnall Highway and its broad median suddenly disappear. The phantom freeway breaks off here and starts up again several blocks later. You'll rejoin it in another 2,000 steps, after a little side trip.

Cross over to the center median on Chandler, whose railroad right-of-way has been converted to a popular walking and biking trail. **Head four blocks east until you get to Hollywood Way. Make a right, so you're heading south.** The next several blocks comprise a quaint commercial district with the kind of shops that are now endangered species in the Valley. A model train shop. A jelly bean store. A baseball card and comic book store. This stretch is also your best chance to

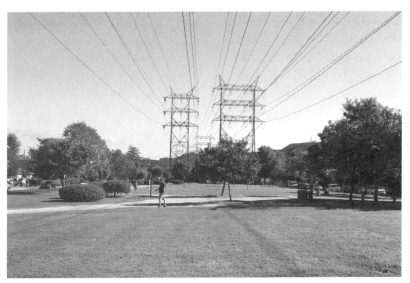

The proposed Whitnall Freeway would have tunneled through the Hollywood Hills in the distance.

fill your stomach. Many of the restaurants have outdoor seating. You can't go wrong with the Cuban sandwiches at Porto's Bakery and Café on the corner of Hollywood and Magnolia Boulevard.

Continue down Hollywood until you cross Clark Avenue. Whitnall Highway will magically reappear on your left. Trek down its southern parkway. Chances are good you'll find a yoga teacher conducting a class with fledgling actors on the grassy median. Resent them for being young, good-looking, and as flexible as Gumby.

After one short block, you'll hit Verdugo Avenue, and the ghost of the superhighway will disappear yet again. This is your turnaround point. **Turn left on Verdugo, then left on Whitnall's northern lanes.**

Head back up Whitnall until you get to Clark again. Turn left, passing Hollywood.

PICNIC OP

The plush grass of the Whitnall Highway median, between Clark Avenue and Verdugo Avenue.

Go three blocks and make a right on Maple Street. Many of the streets in North Hollywood are lined with deciduous trees, ablaze in orange, yellow, and red in the fall. No one will ever mistake this region for

> **EXTRA STEPS**
>
> Whitnall Highway makes one last gasp at relevance another block past Verdugo, between California Street and Fairview Street. The one-block stretch is the only portion without a center median splitting the roadway.

New England, but like much of Los Angeles, there are glimmers of truth in our fallacies. Keep an eye out for the Whitnall Highway corridor after you pass Magnolia. Its power lines pass diagonally overhead.

Turn left on Chandler's cycling/walking path, and 1,400 steps later, you'll pass Cahuenga and encounter a truly hidden gem. On the south side of Chandler, stretching for half a mile, is a series of murals. The subjects range from agriculture to aerospace, from trains to rock 'n' roll—a hodgepodge

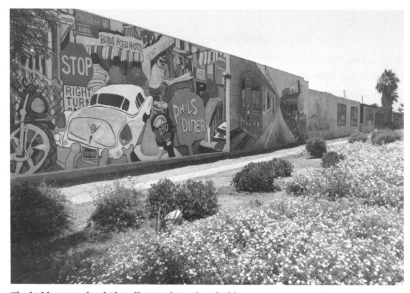

The hidden murals of Chandler Boulevard . . . hidden no more.

of styles painted on the sides of buildings, including corrugated aluminum. The paintings retrace the history of North
Hollywood. Three miles away, the Great Wall of Los Angeles
mural is far better known, but this one scores points for sheer
creativity, use of existing space, and the element of surprise.

The creative streak continues as you **saunter up Satsuma
Avenue** with its array of funky businesses and outdoor art,
including a clock tower that belongs to a prop shop. **At Burbank Boulevard, our route jogs east, then heads north
on Riverton Avenue,** a shady street lined with Chinese elms.
**Take this to Whitnall, then turn left. It's only one more
block to your exit point,** to the freeway that never was.

34

NORTH HOLLYWOOD / TUJUNGA VILLAGE

FROM STATEHOOD TO HOLLYWOOD

This route through two of the Valley's most walkable villages passes through some sacred ground—and we're not just talking about the largest gathering of television stars since a Jerry Lewis telethon, either.

- ■ **TERRAIN:** Flat
- ■ **SURFACE:** Mostly paved
- ■ **FIDO FRIENDLY?:** Yes
- ■ **PARKING:** Street parking near the intersection of Tujunga Avenue and Weddington Street, North Hollywood

Angelenos are by nature apologists. When relatives back East are shivering through ice storms or sweating through sweltering summers, we apologize in dulcet tones for our perfect weather. When the same relatives visit—expecting a garden paradise—we apologize for our bad traffic, lack of good bagels, and marine layers that (horrors!) blot out the sun until early afternoon.

So it is with our history. Rather than embrace the charms of our kitschy past, too often we destroy any landmark that doesn't pass the Old World sniff test. The greater North Hollywood area inverts this pattern . . . somewhat. It makes no apologies for our contributions to pop culture, yet comes up short when it comes to publicizing a location that is of such importance to California, none of this entertainment nonsense would even exist without it!

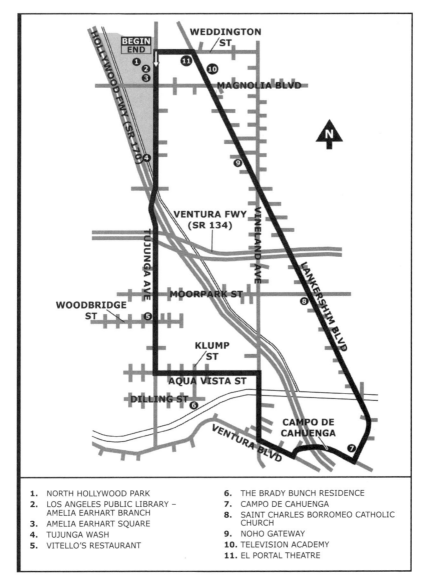

1. NORTH HOLLYWOOD PARK
2. LOS ANGELES PUBLIC LIBRARY – AMELIA EARHART BRANCH
3. AMELIA EARHART SQUARE
4. TUJUNGA WASH
5. VITELLO'S RESTAURANT
6. THE BRADY BUNCH RESIDENCE
7. CAMPO DE CAHUENGA
8. SAINT CHARLES BORROMEO CATHOLIC CHURCH
9. NOHO GATEWAY
10. TELEVISION ACADEMY
11. EL PORTAL THEATRE

From its junction with Weddington Street, cross over to the west side of Tujunga Avenue to North Hollywood Park. Head south, taking a moment to regard the historic 1930 building that is the Amelia Earhart Branch of the Los Angeles Public Library. Earhart lived in North Hollywood for much of her life, and a nearby school is named after her. A statue of the groundbreaking aviator can be found at the intersection of Tujunga and Magnolia Boulevard, known as Amelia Earhart Square.

The park continues past Magnolia, forming a wide greenbelt between Tujunga and the Hollywood Freeway (SR 170) for the next 1,000 steps. As you ramble down the park's decomposed granite walkways, Peter Gabriel's "In Your Eyes" inexplicably fills your head. You crane your neck to the right. Superimposed over the grove of trees, you make out a young man in a brown trench coat holding a boom box above his head. It's Lloyd Dobler, making his stand in the Gen X touchstone film *Say Anything!* Not to be outdone, Pee-wee Herman rides his beloved red bike through the same spot in the opening sequence of *Pee-wee's Big Adventure*. I'd love to see a movie mash-up where Pee-wee rams his two-wheeler into Lloyd, ruining his big romantic moment. "I meant to do that," he'd squawk, untangling himself from Lloyd's baggy trouser legs.

At the south end of the park, pass over Tujunga Wash, which feeds the Los Angeles River a mile south of here. **Continue on Tujunga until you get to Moorpark Street, where you'll enter Tujunga Village**—a plum spot to grab lunch. Despite bountiful boutiques and outdoor cafés, the village is still best known as the site where actor Robert Blake's wife Bonnie Lee Bakley was gunned down in 2001 under suspicious circumstances that many feel pointed to Blake himself. The two had just dined at Vitello's

EXTRA STEPS

It's the story . . . of a house of Bradys. One block south of Aqua Vista is the home used in exterior shots of the 1970s TV show *The Brady Bunch*. Despite some remodeling, it is still instantly recognizable. Head down Klump Street to 11222 Dilling Street (even the address totals eight! Poor Alice—she never quite gets her due).

Restaurant on the corner of Tujunga and Woodbridge Street; she was killed moments later while sitting in their car. In an effort to restore "positive energy," the Italian eatery underwent a renovation and auctioned off the booth where Bakley consumed her last meal.

Two blocks past Vitello's, turn left on Aqua Vista Street and walk 1,000 steps to Vineland Avenue. Go right on Vineland, left on Ventura Boulevard, and left on Campo De Cahuenga, a wide overpass that spans the Hollywood Freeway. On the other side of the bridge, turn left on Lankershim Boulevard.

On your immediate left is a clay-shingled adobe set off from the street and shrouded by trees. While cinematic history is made up the hill at Universal Studios, Campo de Cahuenga's is far more significant. It marks the spot where the U.S. and Mexico signed the Treaty of Cahuenga in 1847, ending the Mexican-American War and paving the way for California statehood in 1850.

As you **walk north on Lankershim,** note the diagonal strip of decorative pavement laid across the boulevard's southbound lanes. It traces the location of the original adobe (the existing one is a replica), whose foundation was unearthed during a subway excavation in 1995. A museum in the adobe holds artifacts from the treaty-signing between Lieutenant Colonel John C. Frémont and General Andrés Pico. In subsequent years, it was learned that Frémont was given secret orders to fan the rebellion that led to California's annexation. Seemingly echoing that secrecy, the museum is closed to the public except for a precious few hours each month. No wonder we don't know much about its history!

After paying tribute to California's birthplace, continue north on Lankershim. On the southwest corner of Moorpark and Lankershim is a Catholic Church erected in 1959. Comedian Bob Hope was a frequent visitor, right up to his well-attended funeral at 100 years old. A sign dedicates the intersection to Bob and his wife Dolores.

Another 1,300 steps up Lankershim brings you to the literal gateway of NoHo—hipspeak for North Hollywood's Arts District. The portal comes in the form of a metal sign extending over Lankershim, a nearly million-dollar project designed to give the region a clearer identity. On the sign, "NoHo" is spelled out against random shapes and film iconography on a lime-green frame. From the moment it went up in 2009, people have been divided: Art or eyesore? Like a lot of creative work, the answer lies in the eye of the beholder.

Half a block north of Magnolia on the east side of the street, head down a driveway leading to a gray and pink courtyard. As you can guess by the fifteen-foot golden Emmy that greets you, this complex is the home of the Television Academy. Next to the Emmy is a bronze statue of Johnny Carson, his gesture imploring you to check out the Hall of Fame Plaza. Dozens of TV legends get their due here, either as busts or life-sized statues. While all the greats

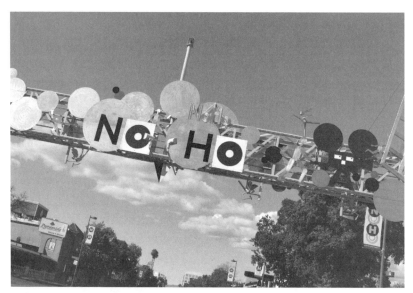

Welcome to the NoHo Arts District.

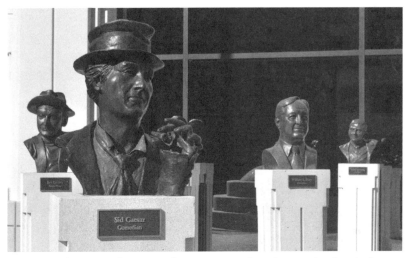

Sculptures of TV greats form an outdoor museum in the Television Academy's plaza.

are represented, a standout is the seated sculpture of Carroll O'Connor and Jean Stapleton from *All in the Family*. Archie Bunker wears a weary expression as he fends off a pestering Edith, perfectly capturing their characters. And where else will you find monuments honoring Jim Henson and his muppets, or William Hanna and Joseph Barbera surrounded by their offspring—Yogi, Fred Flintstone, and Scooby-Doo?

Venture farther up the block to Lankershim and Weddington. Occupying the northwest corner is the El Portal Theatre. Its striking Art Deco marquee dates to 1926, when it debuted as a vaudeville venue. The building sustained severe damage in the 1994 Northridge Earthquake and was threatened with demolition, but thanks to generous supporters it survived and now thrives as a premier playhouse.

From the El Portal, turn left on Weddington. It's one block to your place of origin . . . or 165 years removed and counting, depending on how one looks at it.

35

LAKE VIEW TERRACE

WELL HELLO, HANSEN!

This loop is the perfect escape from the asphalt jungle of the Valley's wide boulevards. But is there really a lake in Lake View Terrace, or is it just another stab at civic boosterism? Here's a hint: don't take this walk after a rainstorm!

- **TERRAIN:** Flat with slight inclines
- **SURFACE:** Paved and unpaved
- **FIDO FRIENDLY?:** Yes
- **PARKING:** Lot at Hansen Dam, Lake View Terrace (from Osborne Street, go east on Dronfield Avenue, turn left after one block, and drive for 0.2 miles; the entrance to the lot will be on your right)
- **NOTE:** Not advisable during rainy season

Quick word association: What comes to mind when someone utters "Lake View Terrace"? It's understandable if your answer is "Rodney King beating." But mere steps from the flashpoint that spawned the 1992 riots is the actual place that puts the "lake" in Lake View Terrace— Hansen Dam, a refuge of recreation and wilderness in the northeastern valley.

After leaving your car in the Osborne Street parking lot, follow the southward flow of pedestrians and bicyclists to the bike path, which has an accompanying dirt trail for walkers. For the next 3,800 steps (almost the entire 2-mile width) you will be walking on top of the dam itself.

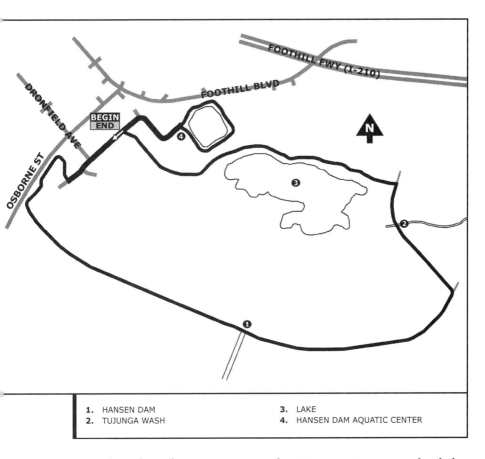

1. HANSEN DAM		**3.** LAKE	
2. TUJUNGA WASH		**4.** HANSEN DAM AQUATIC CENTER	

Like a lot of L.A.'s waterworks, Hansen Dam was built by the U.S. Army Corps of Engineers after the deadly floods of 1938. Giant boulders line its ninety-seven-foot-high earthen walls. The levee lies one mile downstream from the confluence of two rivers that form the Tujunga Wash, which continues through the Valley (and forms the spine of the Valley Village walk) before connecting with the Los Angeles River.

The view on the dam's pathway is pretty spectacular, and there is usually a nice breeze. To your right you'll see the San Fernando Valley; to your left, a riparian flood control basin with miles of trails and lakes backdropped by the San Gabriel and Verdugo Mountains.

Halfway across the dam, the earthen walls give way to a concrete spillway. Like Devil's Gate Dam and Sepulveda Dam, Hansen Dam is designed to simply mitigate water flows. The pathway

> **EXTRA STEPS**
>
> Once you pass over the spillway, descend the dirt incline on the dam's northern face (just past the fence), down into the basin to truly appreciate the spillway gate's Moderne touches.

extends over the spillway, held up by seven elegant arches that epitomize the functional beauty of so many civic projects of the era. Peek over the south end to see Tujunga Wash bursting through concrete sluices on its journey southward.

As you near the eastern edge of the dam, take the wide dirt trail that peels off to the left and descends into the basin. Watch out for horse poop—the trail is popular with equestrians, too! After 800 steps, you'll reach a surprisingly fast-flowing river. This is the Tujunga Wash the way it used to look, in all its unadulterated, naked glory. Looking north, you'll see that the wash is shrouded by natural vegetation. Admire the dive-bombing birds plucking insects off the water. Gazing downriver, you'll find a wide-open area with inviting white sand that looks like the perfect spot for a cabana. Tujunga Beach? No, just sediment brought down from the mountains.

Now the obvious question: How to cross a seven-foot-wide river devoid of bridges? Fortunately, during dry months, it's perfectly shallow and navigable thanks to rocks, logs, and two-by-fours laid across the water by previous hikers. **A hop and a skip and you'll quickly get to the other side.** If it's rained recently, expect to get a little soggy!

From the river, proceed 200 paces until you reach a wide trail to your left. Take this trail, eschewing the main path that heads to the Foothill Freeway (I-210) in the near distance. A tree-lined lake—the basin's centerpiece—will come into view on your left side. Though it has shrunk in size over the years thanks to detritus from the San

Gabriels, the lake is still surprisingly big and pristine—no recreation allowed.

PICNIC OP

Along the northern shore of Hansen Dam's central lake.

Nine hundred steps into this lakeside trail, the path veers left and reaches its closest point to the water. Genuflect to the water's soothing ripples. There really *is* a lake view to be had in Lake View Terrace. Feel your skepticism join the mocking whispers of the wind rustling through the trees.

Now that you're properly chastened, **continue on the trail for a couple hundred steps until you reach the western shore. A smaller dirt trail will appear on your right. Follow this trail for a few hundred steps (with an embankment on your right) until you get to the Osborne parking lot. Exit the lot and turn right on the bike path paralleling an unnamed street. After a sharp right turn, follow the signs into the Hansen Dam Aquatic Center for a little detour.**

The Aquatic Center is actually two lakes. One is a 1.5-acre chlorinated swimming hole that gets packed during the dog days of summer. It can accommodate up to 2,800 swimmers! Next to it is a nine-acre recreational lake where you can fish and take out non-motorized boats.

Amble around the rec lake's 1,000-step loop. Peer into various fishing buckets to find the catches of the day—typically catfish, rainbow trout, and largemouth bass.

Leave the recreational center by returning to the bike path. After 600 steps, the path momentarily disappears, but it picks up again several yards ahead on the other side of the unmarked street. Stay on the bike path for another 500 steps or so, and you'll find yourself back at your car—with a new word association for "Lake View Terrace."

36

BURBANK

BACK IN THE SADDLE

This loop doesn't just look like a horse saddle, it truly is the saddle of Burbank—a charming, older district clinging to its equine roots while serving as the seat upon which a more modern Burbank rests.

- **TERRAIN:** Flat
- **SURFACE:** Paved and unpaved
- **FIDO FRIENDLY?:** Yes, if you bypass Travel Town
- **PARKING:** Lot for Travel Town Railroad at 5200 Zoo Drive, Los Angeles; street parking on Zoo Drive

Like most kids growing up in Los Angeles, my favorite place in the world was Disneyland. But amusement parks cost money, and family visits there were usually limited to once a year. As a result, Plan B saw a lot more action: Travel Town, whose creaky steam engines, rail cars, museum, and miniature railway have been luring train-crazy tykes since the early 1950s.

It's also the starting point for what I like to call Burbank's Saddle. Though it's bisected by the Ventura Freeway (SR 134), the Saddle zone is marked by horses loping down sleepy streets past hay shops and an ice rink, matching Travel Town's timeless innocence, especially when compared to Burbank's more contemporary, northern climes.

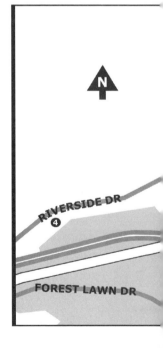

Start by kicking around Travel Town for about 800 steps. Many of the engines are near the entrance. You used to be able to clamber on top of the trains themselves, but walking through them is still cool enough (and less litigious, I suppose).

After leaving Travel Town, exit the parking lot and walk straight onto Zoo Drive. After one short block, turn right on Forest Lawn Drive. You'll see signs to get on the 134 Freeway. Needless to say, do not get on the freeway. Instead, **access the dirt bridle trail on the east side of the street.** The trail ducks beneath an on-ramp for the freeway. Follow the flow of horseback riders and walkers along the

1. TRAVEL TOWN
2. HEADWORKS
3. MARIPOSA EQUESTRIAN BRIDGE
4. ROY E. DISNEY ANIMATION BUILDING
5. PICKWICK DRIVE-IN
   (FORMER LOCATION)
6. PICKWICK RECREATION CENTER
7. LOS ANGELES EQUESTRIAN CENTER
8. BETTE DAVIS PICNIC AREA
9. LOS ANGELES LIVE STEAMERS
   RAILROAD MUSEUM

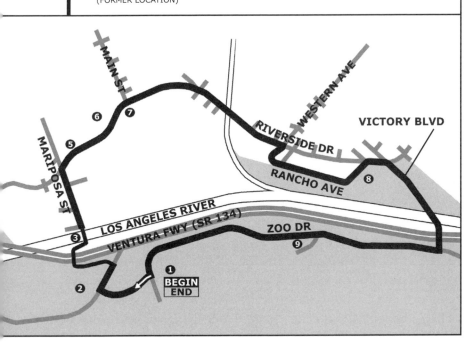

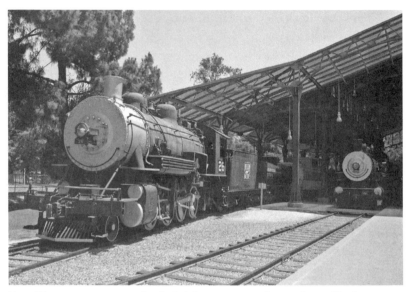

Travel Town never goes out of style. Is it just me, or are these trains smiling?

southern edge of the freeway. The vegetated plot to your left, known as Headworks, is actually subterfuge for two underground reservoirs that store over 100 million gallons of water.

Keep going until the trail cuts through a narrow tunnel. You are now treading under ten lanes of thunderous vehicles, roaring by mere feet above your head. This tunnel connects Griffith Park with the horse stables north of the freeway. Just as important, it's a key wildlife corridor—possibly the route used by P22, the famed puma that took up residence in Griffith Park in 2012.

Emerging on the other side, claustrophobics can now breathe a sigh of relief. Gephyrophobics, it's your turn to steel yourselves. A hundred steps away, the path heads over the rusty Mariposa Equestrian Bridge, which spans the Los Angeles River. While I wouldn't call it unsafe, when was the last time you saw a sign warning you to cross a bridge at your own risk? Another sign stating "Load Limit 6 Horses" also gives pause. As a brigade of horseback riders trots up, you quicken

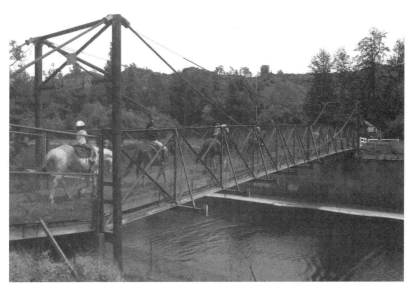

Buttressed by suspension cables, the Mariposa Equestrian Bridge opened only two
years after the Golden Gate Bridge.

your stride over the river, hoping to make it to the other side
before a seventh horse arrives.

**After crossing the bridge, continue north on Maripo-
sa. Turn right on Riverside Drive, staying on the south
side of the street.** On your left, behind a low-lying brick
building, is a massive parking lot. The lot used to be part of
the Pickwick Drive-In, which held up to 800 cars. Mel Brooks's
Blazing Saddles had its premiere there. As a token of its equine
surroundings, the theater set up a "horsepitality bar" for the
movie's stars, who arrived on horseback. In 1989, the drive-in
celebrated its fiftieth anniversary . . . by being torn down. Fortunately, two other hallmarks from that earlier era—a bowling
alley and ice rink—still exist at the Pickwick Recreation Center, a few steps east of here.

On the southwest corner of Riverside and Main Street is
a popular Mexican restaurant—one of the few places to grab
lunch in the vicinity. It's also a famous dinner and margarita

halfway spot for riders renting horses from Sunset Ranch, below the Hollywood Sign. On the southeast corner is the Los Angeles Equestrian Center. Stroll the grounds and watch riders practice their prancing and jumps. You may even be lucky enough to catch an exhibition in the Equidome.

> **EXTRA STEPS**
>
> Horses can go right up to the Roy E. Disney Animation Building—and so can you. Access the equestrian trail just past the bridge and proceed 1,200 steps to the west. Though built in the 1990s, the edifice has a retro-future design. Walt Disney Studios, where Walt once considered building Disneyland, lies across Riverside Drive, which you can follow east back to the main route.

The center boards 400 horses and hosted events for the 1984 Olympics.

The next few blocks take you through the heart of Burbank's Rancho Equestrian District. There's something reassuring about passing by feed stores and horse stables. Every time I pass by the Circle K stables, it reminds me of Brandy—a gentle horse with a sandy mane that my grandmother boarded there for over twenty years. As you wait on street corners for the signal to change, note the two different crosswalk buttons. The higher ones are for horseback riders. I once saw a woman who trained her horse to press the lower button with its nose. This must be what they mean when they talk about horse sense.

Turn right at Western Avenue. After one block, it turns into Rancho Avenue. To your right is the Bette Davis Picnic Area, a long, grassy park shaded by sycamore trees. This is one of the more underutilized parks in the Valley. Bette herself would not stand for this. Please oblige the famous diva by patronizing her rolling acreage for your picnic, if you packed one.

At Riverside Drive, make a right, then another right onto Victory Boulevard. Cross over the L.A. River and Ventura Freeway. At the T-intersection with Zoo Drive,

turn right. Proceed 1,000 steps. On your left is the Los Angeles Live Steamers Railroad

PICNIC OP

Bette Davis Picnic Area, 1850 Riverside Drive.

Museum. Whereas most cities would be lucky to have one rideable miniature railroad, Griffith Park alone is blessed with three. The one here at Live Steamers is the best of the bunch. It's run by train enthusiasts, the most famous of whom was Walt Disney (you didn't think we were done with him yet, did you?). The Steamers' centerpiece is a big red barn that used to belong to Walt himself. It was moved here from his Holmby Hills estate and contains a treasure trove of Disney memorabilia—work benches, toolboxes, early monorail models and his own personal railroad cars. Note that Live Steamers and the barn have limited hours, so check their website before you visit.

From Live Steamers, it's another 1,000 steps back to Travel Town. You have completed the trip around Burbank's Saddle . . . hopefully without the sores.

Overleaf: Kayakers at Marina del Rey.

WESTSIDE

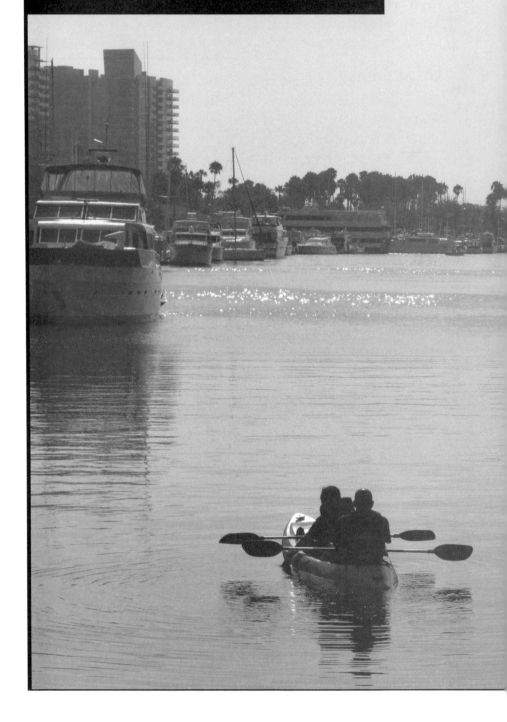

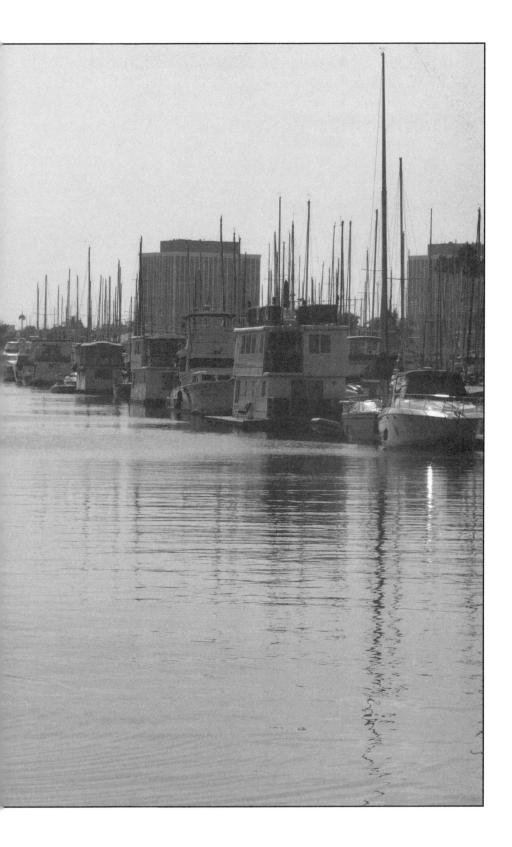

37

SANTA MONICA

FOOTPRINTS OF THE GREAT BANDINI

Mind your P's—Pier, Promenade, and Palisades Park— on this roundabout as we explore Santa Monica's three most walkable and well-known districts in one fell swoop, with a tip o' the hat to the city's real patron saint.

- **TERRAIN:** Flat with stairs and slight inclines
- **SURFACE:** Paved and unpaved
- **FIDO FRIENDLY?:** Yes
- **PARKING:** Street parking on Georgina Avenue, near its intersection with Ocean Avenue in Santa Monica

It would have been very easy for Santa Monica to turn into the next Malibu. Like its elite neighbor up the coast, the city has a postcard-pretty coastline that has long drawn the rich and famous to its shores. But while Malibu residents put up gates and try to block non-residents from their beaches, Santa Monica went the other way, emerging as a progressive outpost that considers the needs of the less-fortunate against a pro-business, pro-tourist environment. Even Marion Davies's former oceanfront mansion has been converted to a community beach house—not surprising for a city once known as "The People's Republic of Santa Monica." As this walk reveals, it's a moniker that didn't happen by accident. It was formed by farsighted visionaries who were intent on weaving the average joe into the fabric of their new hamlet.

From Georgina Avenue, cross Ocean Avenue to

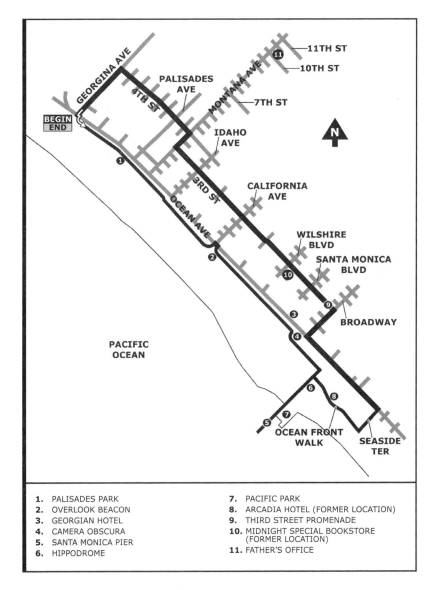

1. PALISADES PARK
2. OVERLOOK BEACON
3. GEORGIAN HOTEL
4. CAMERA OBSCURA
5. SANTA MONICA PIER
6. HIPPODROME
7. PACIFIC PARK
8. ARCADIA HOTEL (FORMER LOCATION)
9. THIRD STREET PROMENADE
10. MIDNIGHT SPECIAL BOOKSTORE (FORMER LOCATION)
11. FATHER'S OFFICE

Palisades Park, a twenty-six-acre greenbelt that extends southward to the Santa Monica Pier. While the pier is, of course, Santa Monica's most timeless landmark, Palisades Park is truly an ode to its past. **Head south along any of the park's decomposed granite walkways. After three**

blocks, you'll reach Palisades Avenue. Turn right on the path that bisects a row of palm trees and leads to a bronze bust in the middle of a rose garden. Meet Arcadia Bandini, the widow of the city's founder, Robert Baker. Along with a business partner, Bandini deeded this acreage to the city in 1892 with the stipulation that it had to be for public use.

Continue south of the rose garden and find a modern wooden sculpture that resembles a giant hollowed-out attic vent. Its official name is *Gestation III*. It changes in appearance as you move around it—a comment on the cycles of the sun.

The next four blocks provide stellar ocean views. Perhaps the best is just past Idaho Avenue, from a beautifully restored, 100-year-old redwood pergola. Then, near California Avenue, there's the Overlook Beacon. It includes a wooden deck and mast that cleverly resembles a boat. A stone monument commemorates the discovery of Santa Monica Bay by Juan Rodriguez Cabrillo on October 8, 1542. A few more steps takes you to a stately limestone bench dedicated to John P. Jones. The U.S. senator came to this spot every day to watch the sunset, prompting him to agree with his business partner, Arcadia Bandini, that these bluffs should be preserved for all to enjoy.

Continue south through Palisades Park. At the foot of Wilshire Boulevard is an eighteen-foot-high Art Deco statue of Santa Monica, the female saint after whom the city is named. Like many monuments in the Southland, it was constructed in the 1930s under Roosevelt's Works Progress Administration.

Just past Santa Monica Boulevard, on the east side of Ocean Avenue, is the historic Georgian Hotel. In the 1920s, it housed a popular speakeasy. These days, it's a regular stop for ghost hunters. Perhaps some of its hooch-hounds got trapped in the hideaway bar?

Proceed another block through the park

> **PICNIC OP**
>
> Palisades Park, in the sitting area of the pergola overlooking the Pacific, two blocks south of Idaho Avenue.

and find the Camera Obscura, a precursor to the modern camera that captures outside images through a hole and projects them onto a screen. This one was built in 1898 and used to sit on the beach. It's now situated in a recreation center. In a rare case of deflation, the price has gone down to use it—once ten cents, it's now free. Simply leave your driver's license on hold for the privilege of spying on unsuspecting passersby.

After 4,000 steps, you'll reach the end of Palisades Park and the entrance to the Santa Monica Pier. Its 1940s sign is a national landmark. The pier is also the official western terminus of Route 66. Look for the "End of the Trail" sign as you **walk down the pier's ramp.**

The first landmark on the left is the pier's historic heart—a Byzantine-style hippodrome, built in 1916. Its original hand-carved carousel horses were designed by Charles Looff, who built the first merry-go-round at Coney Island in 1876. For a while, you could rent apartments above the hippodrome. In *Night Tide*, a movie predating *Splash* by twenty-three years, it's where a maybe-mermaid resides as she dates a pre-hippie Dennis Hopper. Scenes from Best Picture winners *The Sting* and *Forrest Gump* were also filmed here.

Lollygag to the end of the pier—a feast for the senses, as so many SoCal wharfs are. While you could dine at the Third Street Promenade later in this walk, who can pass up greasy fried seafood and French fries from a walk-up counter?

The south end of the pier holds a small amusement park known as Pacific Park. Its name is a wink to Pacific Ocean Park, the sprawling, pier-based entertainment complex between Santa Monica and Venice that opened to much fanfare in 1958. Like a comet, POP shone brightly but briefly, collapsing in a series of fires and mismanagement before finally shuttering less than ten years after it opened.

The Santa Monica Pier almost suffered the same fate as Pacific Ocean Park in the 1970s when it too fell into serious disrepair. Further indignation occurred when a nasty storm in 1983 wiped out its lower deck. Fortunately, smarter heads prevailed and the pier survived through extensive renovation.

To exit the pier, find the stairs east of the hippo-drome, to the right of the automobile ramp. At the base of the stairs, head south on Ocean Front Walk. Look for the sign that says "The Original Location of Muscle Beach—The Birthplace of the Physical Fitness Boom of the Twentieth Century." This *al fresco* exercise area was an-other WPA project, de-signed to keep people of strong mind and body during the Great De-pression. Who knew the government was behind famous he-men Jack LaLanne and Arnold Schwarzenegger, two of Muscle Beach's frequent visitors? Though you will still find exercise equipment here, Muscle Beach moved to Venice Beach in 1959.

STEPPING BACK

Out of the ashes of Pacific Ocean Park rose the Z-Boys of Dogtown—the nickname given to the renegade surfers who threaded the pier's crumbling pilings and birthed the surfing and skateboarding culture co-opted by America's youth in the 1970s. Their exploits were captured in a documentary and a feature film in the early 2000s.

You'll also notice a walkway named Arcadia Terrace that intersects Ocean Front Walk. A massive Victorian hotel once stood on the left. Considered the grandest inn in the South-land when it opened in 1887, the Arcadia Hotel—there's our friend Arcadia, again—included a rollercoaster that took guests down to the sand. It's also where a liquored-up Colonel Griffith of Griffith Park fame shot his wife in the eye in 1903. She fell two stories but miraculously lived. Like something out of a Betty Boop cartoon, an awning cushioned her fall.

Continue along Ocean Front for 300 steps until you reach a parking lot just south of a cream-colored res-idential building. Pass through the lot and return to Ocean Avenue via Seaside Terrace, a pedestrian-on-ly walkway. Head north on Ocean, then turn right on

Broadway. After two blocks, you'll reach the entrance to the Third Street Promenade on your left.

If the pier and Palisades Park represent its past, nothing captures Santa Monica's present quite like its Promenade. Since its christening in 1989, it's been a rousing success. With apartments stacked above stores and movie theaters, it reintroduced the mixed-use concept to Angelenos—something that had fallen out of favor but is now standard everywhere. Originally, the promenade was known as the Santa Monica Mall (it's featured in *Pee-wee's Big Adventure*). But within a few years of its 1965 opening, homeless people often outnumbered pedestrians. My most vivid childhood memory from that era: a dead rat floating in one of its broken water fountains.

While no one misses the danger element, some residents feel that high rents have made the mall too sanitized, with upscale stores and restaurants muscling out smaller independents that brought more character. One thing that has remained constant, however, are the old buildings' Art Deco and Streamline Moderne facades. Look above the doorway at 1318 3rd Street. Sandwiched between the bricks is a frieze of books, a spectral reminder of its former occupant, the Midnight Special bookstore.

After three blocks, the Promenade ends at Wilshire. Keep going north for 1,000 steps, into Santa Monica's residential area, and turn right on Montana Avenue. After one block, make a left on 4th Street.

Follow 4th to Georgina and turn left. It's one long block back to its junction with Ocean Avenue. The street itself is a final testament to the legacy of Arcadia Bandini, who died in her home on Ocean Avenue in 1912.

EXTRA STEPS

For a boutiquey detour, take Montana Avenue for several blocks east, starting at 7th Street. The original Father's Office, which essentially launched L.A.'s gastropub movement, can be found between 10th and 11th Streets.

38

PACIFIC PALISADES

A STROLL FOR THE SOUL

Sometimes you just need to slow down and feed your inner "chi," whether it's a hike among nature, a quiet visit to a lakeside shrine, or a trip to an art museum. Why not do all three in Pali? Your body and mind will thank you later.

- **TERRAIN:** Flat with stairs and several inclines, including one short, steep one
- **SURFACE:** Paved and unpaved
- **FIDO FRIENDLY?:** No (not allowed at the Self-Realization Fellowship Lake Shrine or the Getty Villa)
- **PARKING:** Street parking on Los Liones Drive near its intersection with Tramonto Drive, one block west of Sunset Boulevard, Pacific Palisades
- **NOTE:** Advance reservations required for the Getty Villa

Most people associate Pacific Palisades with its charming village and Will Rogers State Historic Park, which includes hiking trails and a polo field that were once part of the entertainer's estate. Farther west on Sunset Boulevard, however, is where you'll find the Palisades' contemplative center. In a fitting coincidence, even its nickname—Pali—is the same word for an ancient Eastern language that laid the groundwork for the earliest Buddhist scripture.

Start with a little warm-up along a nature trail to get your heart pumping. From its intersection with Tramonto Drive, look for the sign on the east side of Los Liones Drive that reads "Topanga State Park: Los Liones Can-

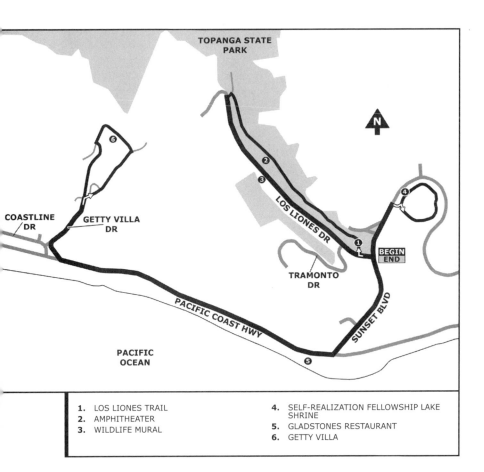

1. LOS LIONES TRAIL
2. AMPHITHEATER
3. WILDLIFE MURAL
4. SELF-REALIZATION FELLOWSHIP LAKE SHRINE
5. GLADSTONES RESTAURANT
6. GETTY VILLA

yon Entrance." **Access the nature trail,** which is mostly flat and includes a footbridge that goes over a seasonal stream. Informational signs point out various flora and fauna.

After 1,000 steps, the trail will swing left and head into the wilds of 9,000-acre Topanga State Park. Do not continue on it! Instead, find the metal fence to your left and walk through the stone-and-wood threshold. Next, head through the parking lot and down Los Liones Drive.

Halfway down the street is a mural that depicts local wildlife in meticulous detail: a blue jay holds a toyon berry in its beak while hummingbirds suck nectar from red salvia.

Anchoring the mural at
the wall's highest point
are a pair of mountain
lions gazing directly at
you, reminders that Los
Liones is, after all, named
after the park's apex predators.

PICNIC OP

The small outdoor amphitheater
in Topanga State Park, about 700
steps from the Sunset Boulevard
trailhead.

Stay on Los Liones until you get to Sunset Boulevard.
Observe the flat-faced boulder at the northwest corner of the
intersection, next to a fire station. Its rusty 1959 plaque is dedicated to the native peoples who first lived here. **Cross Sunset
at the crosswalk and turn left. Just past a residential
building is a driveway leading to the Self-Realization
Fellowship Lake Shrine.** (To visit the fellowship's headquarters, flip to the Highland Park/Mount Washington walk.)
Pass under the archway and onto the grounds.

The shrine is named after its cornerstone, Lake Santa Ynez,
supposedly the only natural spring-fed lake in Los Angeles.
The ten-acre site once provided shelter from the glare of celebrity for George Harrison and even Elvis Presley, who came
here looking for answers that could not be solved by the magical pull of his white jumpsuits. While the landscape is dominated by a sixteenth-century Dutch windmill and the Golden
Lotus Archway, the shrine is laid out in a way that invites discovery. As you wander its pathways, hidden ornaments unfurl
before you like the petals of a lotus blossom. Among them: a
shrine that contains ashes from Mahatma Gandhi.

Having rejuvenated your spirit with a boost from India,
you're ready to move on to more Western inspirations. **Exit
the Lake Shrine through the same driveway from which
you entered. Turn left on Sunset and log 800 steps to the
Pacific Coast Highway.** If you're feeling hungry, Gladstones
Restaurant at the corner of Sunset and PCH is a seafood staple. However, it's also a bit of a scene. Remember, you're riding a spiritual plane. Perhaps you'll want to dine in the quiet

café at your final destination—the Getty Villa.

To get to the Getty, walk west on PCH (staying on the south sidewalk and shoulder, with the ocean on your left). As you approach 1,400 highway steps, look for the large retaining wall on the north side of the street. The entrance to the Getty Villa is just past that wall. Cross Coastline Drive at the corner, and hoof it up the museum's hilly driveway—Getty Villa Drive. A sign declares, "Parking: $15." See? You're already saving money by walking.

The iconic Getty Center in Brentwood may get more attention, but this Getty has been around much longer. Admission is free for both, with one key difference: the Getty Villa requires advance reservations, so be sure to secure a time through their website before this walk!

At the top of the hill you'll find immaculate gardens that would make Caesar himself preen in triumph. A 220-foot-long reflecting pool is buttressed by hedge-lined walkways. Peristyles jut out from a replica of an ancient Roman country villa. The grounds contain over 300 plants and species from the Mediterranean, accented by bronze sculptures, fountains, and arbors. Inside the galleries are 44,000 antiquities from ancient Greece and Rome covering 7,000 years.

The museum owes its existence to the fact that its benefactor, J. Paul Getty, was a bit of a hoarder. Running out of room in his Pacific Palisades mansion to keep his Classical collectibles, the billionaire opened this museum in 1974 to ensure their proper storage.

After drinking in the magnificent view of the Pacific Ocean, leave the villa by heading back down the driveway and retracing your steps back to Los Liones Drive. If you're still waiting to exhale, now would be a good time to do it.

39

VENICE

CHANNELING ABBOT KINNEY

Sorry, Harry Perry—this walk through Venice forgoes the boardwalk, focusing instead on the neighborhood's famed canals. The first half retraces the ones that used to exist. The second half visits those that are still flourishing, with a detour to one of the last lagoons in Los Angeles.

- **TERRAIN:** Flat
- **SURFACE:** Paved and unpaved
- **FIDO FRIENDLY?:** Yes
- **PARKING:** Lot at 2150 Dell Avenue, between N. Venice Boulevard and S. Venice Boulevard, Venice; street parking is also available on Venice Boulevard

Weirdness is in Venice's DNA. Ever since developer Abbot Kinney declared that he would recreate Venice, Italy, out of beachfront swampland in 1904, the community has not been short on characters . . . or character. You can see it not just in the gypsy with the live snake scarf who will read you poetry for a dollar, but in the odd-angled streets east of Pacific Avenue. For it is here that Kinney's original canals lie dormant under coffins of striped blacktop. So hop into your imaginary gondola as we glide through the former waterway network.

Start at the intersection of N. Venice Boulevard and Dell Avenue. Head west on N. Venice Boulevard until it intersects Canal Street. Spy the painted portrait of a gaunt,

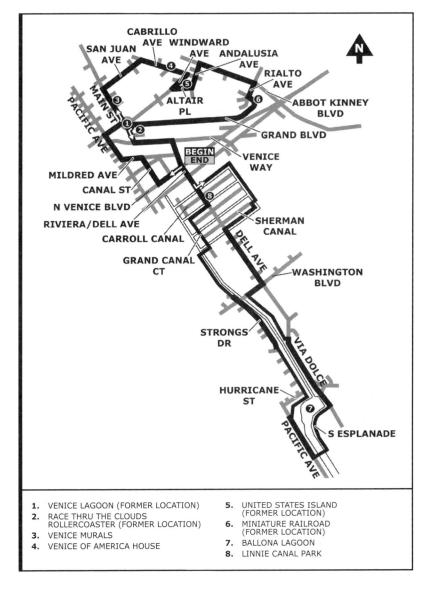

1. VENICE LAGOON (FORMER LOCATION)
2. RACE THRU THE CLOUDS ROLLERCOASTER (FORMER LOCATION)
3. VENICE MURALS
4. VENICE OF AMERICA HOUSE
5. UNITED STATES ISLAND (FORMER LOCATION)
6. MINIATURE RAILROAD (FORMER LOCATION)
7. BALLONA LAGOON
8. LINNIE CANAL PARK

bearded man peeking out from behind a brick building just west of Pacific Avenue. This is Abbot Kinney, his specter presiding over this pivotal junction—a crossroads in Venice's history. On the left side of the street is an old canal, dead-ending here at Venice Boulevard. The truncated channel used to flow under the boulevard, leading to other canals on your right. Their deteriorating state coincided with the rise of automobiles, prompting the city of Los Angeles to convert the northern waterways to streets shortly after annexing Venice in 1926.

Turn right on Canal Street, which retraces the former *actual* canal for a block and a half. **Go left on Mildred Avenue, then right on Pacific** (formerly Trolley Way). At the corner of Pacific and Windward Avenue are a series of buildings with arches, holdouts of the colonnade architecture that once dominated the region. This intersection famously doubled as Tijuana in the long opening tracking shot of Orson Welles's *Touch of Evil.*

Turn right on Windward. In one block, you'll arrive at the Venice Lagoon—or what became of it. Now an uninspiring traffic circle, the lagoon once fed three different canals that now extend outward as streets. Pause long enough, though, and you'll hear the faint but shrill screams of ghost riders. They come from the right of the traffic circle, where the Race Thru the Clouds rollercoaster stood from 1911 to 1923. The nearly mile-long ride was a cornerstone of Kinney's fully realized plans to create a Coney Island of the West. Talk about an overachiever.

Follow the traffic circle counterclockwise. Check out the commercial building at the corner of Main Street and Grand Boulevard. Its curved façade is a visual homage to the former rollercoaster.

Continue around the circle and then head north on Main, once a north-south waterway known as Coral Canal. Look for a couple of cool murals on the right. The first is a snapshot of Venice in its heyday that bends around the corner of Main and Market Street. The other, at Main and Horizon Avenue, features Dennis Hopper on his motorcycle in *Easy Rider.* A longtime Venice resident with a studio nearby, the actor/painter epitomized Venice's rebellious streak.

Following the old Coral Canal route (Main Street), turn right at San Juan Avenue, formerly San Juan Canal. **Continue on San Juan until it turns into Cabrillo Avenue** (née Cabrillo Canal). Cabrillo held the distinction of being the farthest canal from the ocean. Many of the homes here date back to that aqueous age, most famously the so-called Venice of America House at 1223 Cabrillo, built by Abbot Kinney himself in 1906. It's the oldest house in Venice.

While living on a canal might be novel, only one thing can beat it: living on an *island* surrounded by canals. That's exactly what you'll find a block past Kinney's place. **After turning right on Windward Avenue/Canal,** you'll come to a neat row of pastel-colored bungalows on the left. These are the descendents of what used to be United States Island, bounded by Cabrillo, Windward, and Altair Canals. Each house on the island was named after a U.S. state.

Next, go left on Altair, left on Andalusia Avenue, and then right on Abbot Kinney Boulevard. Kinney's eponymous street has traded in its head shops to become the Westside's hipper answer to Rodeo Drive, a transformation that would probably make the known populist roll over in his grave. No matter—this is one of the most eclectic retail sections of Los Angeles and a fun place to people-watch while you treat yourself to an overpriced meal.

Following Abbot Kinney east, turn right on Rialto Avenue, then left on Grand. The street retraces the path of the former Grand Canal. To your left, where residential complexes now stand, was once a Miniature Railroad that was a popular attraction.

Follow Grand back to the former Venice Lagoon. Grand Canal used to extend south via Main Street, leading to additional canals south of Venice Boulevard that still exist. You can thank the Great Depression for that—the city ran out of money to fill them in with concrete. To get to these living dinosaurs, **go left on Main, left on Venice Way, and right on**

Riviera Avenue, which turns into Dell Avenue. From Dell, turn left at the "Do Not Enter" sign just before the bridge that passes over Carroll Canal. Access the walkway along Carroll, the up-

permost canal of the remaining grid of six. Ironically, the six survivors weren't built by Kinney, but by a syndicate called the Short Line Beach Company.

Stay on the path as it turns south and becomes the Eastern Canal walkway, admiring the venerable Cape Cod-type mansion at the canals' confluence. Staying on Eastern Canal, you'll pass two bridges on your right that are prime picture spots. Because there are no cars, this is one of the quietest residential areas in Los Angeles.

Turn right at the third footbridge. Make a left on the walkway, following it as it runs along Sherman Canal, the southernmost channel. When you reach Dell again, turn left. Follow it to Washington Boulevard and cross the street.

Head west on Washington for about 150 steps and look for the dirt pathway to the left, behind the three-story residential building at 311 Washington. Access this pathway, which mirrors Grand Canal.

Three hundred steps in, the walkway will curve left and let out onto a sidewalk for Via Dolce. Turn right. After 400 steps, find the dirt walkway known as

South Esplanade. It fronts a coastal wetland known as Ballona Lagoon. The marshland supports over eighty-six types of plants and serves over sixty species of birds along the Pacific Flyway. Interpretive placards are strategically placed along its perimeter.

The walkway quickly bends to the left around a building. Once it does, **follow the footbridge on your right that heads over the lagoon and brings you to Pacific Avenue. Turn right, following the sidewalk adjacent to the lagoon.** At Jib Street, the pathway leaves Pacific, curving around a utility station before returning you to Washington.

Cross Washington and continue along the west bank of Grand Canal. You will find yourself back in the historic canal district.

> **EXTRA STEPS**
>
> To circumnavigate the entire Ballona Lagoon, bypass the footbridge and tread 1,200 more steps to Via Marina. Turn right and follow the path northward. Another 1,200 steps will deposit you on the other side of the footbridge on Pacific Avenue.

Cross over the first bridge you get to, turn left, then hopscotch over the next three bridges and canals via Grand Canal Court. After the third bridge, turn right on Carroll Canal Court. At Dell Avenue, you'll encounter a pocket park (Linnie Canal Park) that has a pint-sized canal bridge for the kiddies.

Turn left on Dell, which will take you back to S. Venice Boulevard. Mr. Kinney's dream of a fully realized "Venice West" didn't last much beyond his lifetime. But he was just crazy enough to give it a good go—conventions be damned—and isn't that what modern-day Venice is still all about?

40

MARINA DEL REY

WALKING BY THE DOCK OF THE BAY

The nation's largest man-made, small-craft harbor can accommodate over 6,000 boats. And while it sometimes takes some doing to find it, its waterfront has miles of walkways to take in the views—boat shoes not required.

■ **TERRAIN:** Flat
■ **SURFACE:** Paved
■ **FIDO FRIENDLY?:** Yes
■ **PARKING:** Lot 9, 14110 Palawan Way, Marina del Rey

Marina del Rey is a relative latecomer to the Los Angeles County scene. Born in the '60s but coming of age in the '70s, its cylindrical high-rise condos, cheesy nightclubs, and access to yachts on which to "partay" quickly earned it a reputation as a bachelor's paradise. But times change, and like some of its first-generation residents, the marina seems to be undergoing a kind of midlife crisis, unsure of what it wants to be next. Moreover, much of its waterfront is frustratingly inaccessible to the public, bearing the scars of post-World War II city planning in which the car was king. But with a little creativity, you can enjoy a nice up-and-back

STEPPING BACK

In its previous, untamed life, Marina del Rey was a giant salt marsh, fed by Ballona Creek to the south. Before the pleasure crafts arrived, pleasure hunters flocked to the estuary to shoot ducks.

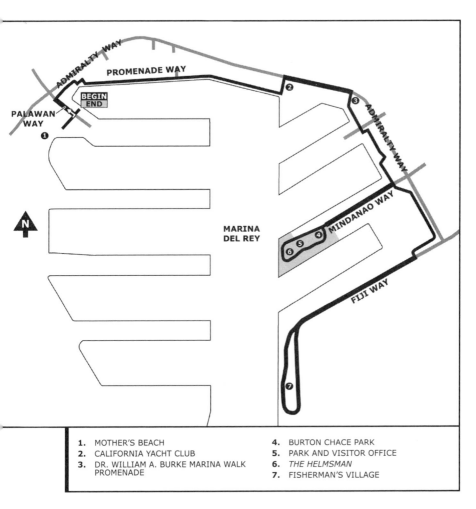

1. MOTHER'S BEACH
2. CALIFORNIA YACHT CLUB
3. DR. WILLIAM A. BURKE MARINA WALK
   PROMENADE
4. BURTON CHACE PARK
5. PARK AND VISITOR OFFICE
6. *THE HELMSMAN*
7. FISHERMAN'S VILLAGE

route that takes in much of this 824-acre engineering marvel.

Leave Parking Lot 9 via its driveway and walk to the other side of Palawan Way to access Mother's Beach, a roped-off inlet with sandy shores that provides the only beachfront in the marina. The lagoon is ideal not just for families, but also for windsurfers, kayakers, and others seeking calm ocean waters. Make a mental note to add "learn stand-up paddleboarding" to your to-do list.

Return to Lot 9. The east side of the lot abuts one of the marina's eight harbor basins. **Turn left and find the globes of light that mark the beginning of Promenade Way,** a pedestrian path that starts next to Killer Shrimp restaurant. **Turn right on Promenade** and enjoy the views (and names) of the boats in their slips. While many of the boats are for pleasure, others double as homes. The county allows only five percent liveaboards, with a waiting list that rivals that of replacement organ recipients. Note the groovy wave pattern on the metal fence that separates the path from the marina. On your left are several restaurants with outdoor seating offering elevated harbor views. Admire the patrons sipping their mimosas, but only for a fleeting moment; you're burning calories while they're adding them.

Stay on Promenade Way for 1,200 steps. At that point, you'll come to the final restaurant, a rambunctious staple known as Tony P's Dockside Grill. The walkway ends abruptly at a white metal gate flanked by barbed wire. A no-nonsense sign will inform you that beyond those doors lies the private California Yacht Club and that you are being videotaped. **Press on through Tony P's parking lot, making a right on the sidewalk alongside Admiralty Way.**

Just past the library, find the sign at the parking lot entrance (excuse all the parking lots, but this is L.A.) that says "Dr. William A. Burke Marina Walk Promenade," named after a prominent California Coastal Commissioner. The marina-adjacent walkway picks up again here, mirroring a bike path. **Take it to Mindanao Way,** one of many streets around here named after islands in the Pacific or the Philippines. **Turn right on Mindanao, which runs into Burton Chace Park.**

Reaching into the harbor like an outstretched finger, the little-known park contains some quirky features dreamed up by county designers. First, you'll be greeted by a beautifully tiled water fountain and a tribute to the "Father of the Marina," Burton W. Chace, whose rendering bears an uncanny

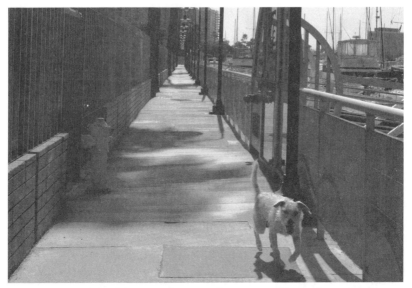

Porter enjoys the bayside breezes of Promenade Way . . . and, no doubt, its fire hydrants.

resemblance to former UCLA demigod John Wooden. As the sign explains, the former county

PICNIC OP

Burton Chace Park, 13650 Mindanao Way.

supervisor is credited for converting "these formerly mosquito-infested mudflats into the now world-renowned marina." Next, enter the Park and Visitor Office and take in the historical photos charting the origins of Marina del Rey under the gently reprimanding heading: "Marina del Rey: It didn't just happen."

Head south and notice a public restroom with porthole windows, which probably seemed like a good idea at the time. Next to the restroom is a small, enclosed dirt lot—about five by ten feet—with one lonely tree. Improbably, a sign says "Dog Run." If this isn't the smallest dog run in the world, I'd like to know what is. I let Porter in here and he just looked at me and whimpered, as if I had just locked him in solitary confinement. Just west of the restroom is another dog area, this one only slightly bigger. I will say this: the harbor views are fantastic, making this dog park the canine equivalent of those microstudios in Manhattan.

Before leaving the park, be sure to take in the impressive bronze statue on the western promontory. It depicts a sea captain in a hooded raincoat and knee-high galoshes braving a storm at sea. If you think he looks like the bearded skipper on the package of Gorton's Fish Sticks, you're not alone. *The Helmsman* used to front the old Helms Bakery in Culver City. A local yacht club donated a new steering wheel. Hey, maybe those guys are all right after all!

Exit the park and retrace your steps on Mindanao Way. Turn right at the corner of Mindanao and Admiralty. After one block, hang another right on Fiji Way. A sign will direct you to Fisherman's Village. In another 1,000 steps, the road curves and you'll see the "Fisherman's Village Entrance" sign directing you into—uh-

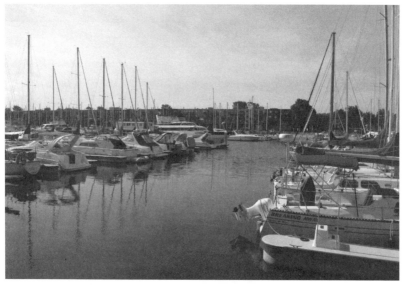

Just another day in paradise.

huh—a parking lot. Cut through the lot and explore the quaint Cape Cod-inspired village, which offers several eateries and an ice cream stand. Behind it is a seaside promenade whose docks offer parasailing, sportfishing, even cruises to Catalina Island. This is a wonderful place to get some food to go and lazily watch the boats drift by as seagulls caw overhead.

It should be noted that the county is planning a complete overhaul of Fisherman's Village, which may even be in motion by the time you read this. Admittedly, its faux lighthouse and shopworn buildings could use some sprucing up. But while the '60s may not have been a good time for pedestrians, it *was* still of an era when L.A. embraced playful architecture. Hopefully any reimagining of Fisherman's Village preserves its offbeat origins. At the very least, word has it that the lighthouse will be spared.

Just past the lighthouse, the village comes to an end. Make a left—through a parking lot—and stride back to Mother's Beach. You can obviously bypass Chace Park when you do . . . unless you feel like snickering at that giant fish stick statue again.

41

PLAYA DEL REY

A BUNCH OF BALLONA

Ballona Creek, Ballona Sand Dunes, and Ballona Wetlands form the basis of this beach-adjacent walk through a trolleyless town that's a real Playa.

- **TERRAIN:** Flat with two moderate inclines
- **SURFACE:** Paved and unpaved
- **FIDO FRIENDLY?:** Yes
- **PARKING:** Lot for Del Rey Lagoon Park, 6660 Esplanade, Playa del Rey; more lots on Pacific Avenue; street parking also available

Playa del Rey is Spanish for "Beach of the King," but its grandiose name belies a small, mellow coastal hood that has been spared from the tsunami of Westside encroachment. Much of that is due to geography. Playa del Rey is hemmed in by the LAX runway to the south, protected wetlands to the east, Marina del Rey to the north, and the Pacific Ocean to the west.

Begin this walk at Del Rey Lagoon Park. Its marshland can be traced to 1870, when a syndicate attempted to dredge Santa Monica Bay to create a shipping port. Their plans did not quite pan out, but it did yield the park's lovely lagoon, created by accidental flooding.

Exit the park by going south on Esplanade. Just east of its junction with Culver Boulevard is a legendary

PICNIC OP

Del Rey Lagoon Park, between Pacific Avenue and Esplanade.

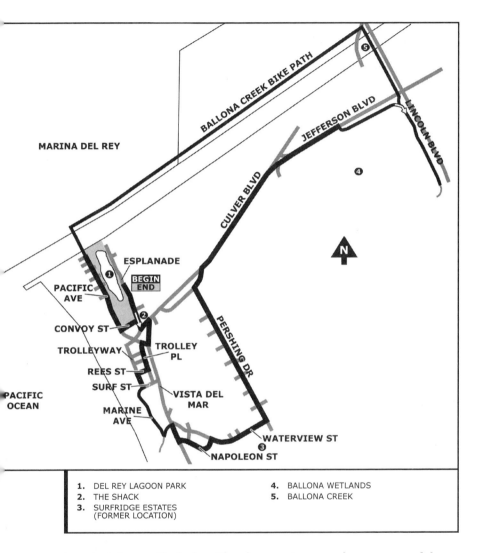

1. DEL REY LAGOON PARK
2. THE SHACK
3. SURFRIDGE ESTATES
   (FORMER LOCATION)
4. BALLONA WETLANDS
5. BALLONA CREEK

lunch joint called the Shack, serving up burgers and beer (hint, hint) since 1972.

From the Shack, turn right on Vista Del Mar. Welcome to the Jungle, a four-block section whose name allegedly derives from the overgrowth of foliage spilling onto the sidewalks. This area used to be served by trolleys, and to this day is bookended by two streets named Trolley Place and

Trolleyway.

Head south on Trolley Place and turn right on either Fowling, Rees, or Sunridge to get to Trolleyway. Go left on Trolleyway and follow it to Surf Street. Take the bike/pedestrian path on your right and proceed south for about 150 feet to the end of a building. At that point, turn left onto another pathway known as Marine Avenue. The beach here is nice and wide and one of the least frequented in L.A.

Four hundred steps later, locate the series of dirt trails to your left that climb a short incline. Traipse up one of the pathways and make a right onto Vista Del Mar. After one block, cross over to Napoleon Street, a sloped street heading away from the beach.

Fenced off to your right are dying palm trees lining empty streets and vacant, weedy lots. The endangered El Segundo Blue Butterfly is about the only resident left in Surfridge Estates, once one of L.A.'s most desirable beachfront neighborhoods ("Rivaling the Romantic Seaside Settings of Yesterday!" boasted promotional signs, somewhat awkwardly). Cecil B. DeMille, Mel Blanc, and Carmen Miranda were among those who called it home. Beginning in the mid-'60s, 822 homes were torn down due to the airport's expansion and noise concerns, leaving behind this haunting, post-cataclysmic landscape. To view its northern boundary, **turn right on Waterview Street, which ends at a T-intersection with Pershing Drive.**

Go left on Pershing. After 1,600 steps, turn right at the T-intersection, bearing right at the bottom of the hill onto Culver Boulevard. The street will take you through a wide-open expanse of protected sand dunes. **Continue east when you reach Jefferson Boulevard.** To your right, you'll see the Ballona Wetlands, an ecological reserve harboring one of the last remaining marshes in Los Angeles. Unfortunately, the trail around it is off-limits unless accompanied by guided tour. But as you walk along Jefferson's dirt pathway, you can still observe the wetlands and the herons, egrets, and other birds that make it their home.

When you get to Lincoln Boulevard, turn right, where the perimeter trail contin-

ues for another 1,000 steps. Sadly, these 640 acres represent only one-third of the original Ballona Wetlands, but given the threat of development that has loomed over this valuable land throughout the years, score this one a tie, which is better than a total loss.

Turn around on Lincoln and leave the marsh by crossing Jefferson. Stay on the west side of Lincoln, which remains a dirt path. Six hundred steps past Jefferson, cross over Ballona Creek. Just past the overpass, find the trail to your left that leads to the bike-and-pedestrian path—a straight shot toward the ocean alongside Ballona Creek, which, like many L.A. waterways, used to be au naturel until it was clothed in concrete to mitigate flooding.

At the path's 1,600-step mark, a second route veers off toward Fisherman's Village (see the Marina del Rey walk). Continue past this cutoff. The path now navigates a narrow jetty. Take a moment to appreciate your surroundings: Ballona Creek to your left, sail boats sluicing the marina to your right, and ocean breezes tickling your face. This is arguably the prettiest stretch of bikeway in the entire city.

As you get closer to the mouth of the marina, follow the flow of human traffic over the bridge to the left that spans Ballona Creek. Welcome back to Del Rey Lagoon Park, where your journey to the land of Ballona began.

42

WEST LOS ANGELES

FREEDOM WALK

Imagine walking 10,000 steps through the heart of West L.A. and encountering zero traffic, a couple of nature sanctuaries, and plenty of green space that invites introspection. Now stop imagining and thank a veteran for the opportunity.

- **TERRAIN:** Flat with stairs
- **SURFACE:** Paved
- **FIDO FRIENDLY?:** No (not allowed on cemetery grounds)
- **PARKING:** Lot for Los Angeles National Cemetery, 950 Sepulveda Boulevard, Los Angeles (from Sepulveda, go east on Constitution Avenue; turn right into the lot)

Like many reading this, I've had loved ones who served in the armed forces. My father enlisted in World War II and became a bombardier, slated for combat in the Pacific until a medical emergency knocked him out of commission. Growing up on L.A.'s Westside, I'm embarrassed to admit that I never gave much thought to the veterans cemetery next to Westwood or the adjacent Department of Veterans Affairs grounds. Researching this walk forced me to take a closer look at both, heightening my appreciation for the sacrifices made by generations of Americans dating back to the Civil War.

This pilgrimage of sorts starts at the Los Angeles National Cemetery. Opened in 1889, it contains 86,000 internments across 114 acres. **From the parking lot, cross over to the north side of Constitution Avenue, to the Spanish Revival-influenced Bob Hope Veterans Chapel.** No

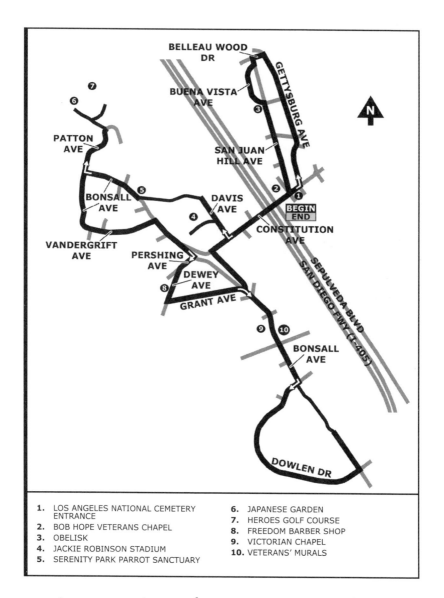

1. LOS ANGELES NATIONAL CEMETERY
   ENTRANCE
2. BOB HOPE VETERANS CHAPEL
3. OBELISK
4. JACKIE ROBINSON STADIUM
5. SERENITY PARK PARROT SANCTUARY

6. JAPANESE GARDEN
7. HEROES GOLF COURSE
8. FREEDOM BARBER SHOP
9. VICTORIAN CHAPEL
10. VETERANS' MURALS

prominent entertainer made more trips to America's overseas troops than Hope. On his ninety-ninth birthday, "GI Bob" was honored with a plaque that shows him donning a USO badge.

Return to Constitution and head east, turning left on Gettysburg Avenue. Don't be surprised if you're the only

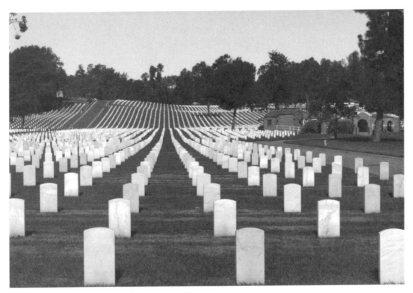

The headstones of Los Angeles National Cemetery.

person here. Walking in heavy silence amidst neatly aligned rows of headstones is a sobering experience.

As Gettysburg starts to curve, it leads to two brick buildings dating back to the WPA days—a pergola and columbarium. Go inside the latter and view the displays of military uniforms, as well as hundreds of urns in the walls. Just south of these structures is a cast-zinc figure of a Union soldier from 1896.

Follow Gettysburg up a small hill to Belleau Wood Drive. Make a left, then another left on San Juan Hill Avenue. Turn right on Buena Vista Avenue, which has two turnouts holding Union Army caissons—wooden carts designed for carrying artillery and dead bodies.

Where Buena Vista reconnects with San Juan Hill, you'll find a granite obelisk erected in memory of fallen soldiers. The monument is perched on a bluff with sweeping views of the gravestones.

Descend San Juan Hill and exit the cemetery via Constitution. By the time you leave the grounds, you'll have accumulated 2,000 steps. **Cross under the San Diego Freeway (I-405) to the intersection of Constitution and Davis Avenue.** You will find yourself on Veterans Administration property, some 600 acres of unincorporated land providing medical and social services for war veterans. As the landlord, Uncle Sam also rents out space to tenants like UCLA. The university's baseball team plays at Jackie Robinson Stadium, to your right.

Find the stairs with yellow hand rails, just past the parking lot, and take them up to the concourse, which is usually open. (During baseball season, you can watch the players practice on the field.) Admire the statue of Jackie Robinson, a UCLA alumnus who, of course, also broke baseball's color barrier. Remind yourself to come back and catch a game, where a field-level seat can be had for less than the price of a single beer at Dodger Stadium!

Retrace your steps down the stairs and continue eastward through the parking lot, turning left on Davis. The street ends at a parking lot for a nursery. To its left is a driveway that skirts the outfield of the stadium. Head down this driveway (fantasizing about what it would be like to play center field for the Bruins) until you hear loud squawking. That's the first audible sign that you're entering the ironically named Serenity Park Parrot Sanctuary, one of L.A.'s best-kept secrets. The complex is home to a dozen or so parrots who like to greet you with "hellos" as you approach their aviaries. It's lovingly maintained by veterans who are happy to introduce you to their feathered chums, including one who is partial to warbling the words to "Hello, Dolly!"

To depart, ascend the short pathway just north of the sanctuary, or the one that leads out of the parking lot. Both will take you to Bonsall Avenue. Head north on Bonsall—passing Patton Avenue—until you hit a T-intersection. Turn right here, onto another section of Patton Avenue.

The quietude on campus in strangely discomfiting in the middle of an otherwise boisterous metropolis. The sleepy buildings date back decades, with signs alluding to their primary purposes. According to the Los Angeles Conservancy, nearly forty percent of the structures are considered historic, many either vacant or in need of renovation. What to do with them (privatize them? Convert to homeless housing?) is a source of constant debate.

After 200 steps, Patton leads to a fork. Take the driveway on the left that's marked "Japanese Garden." This is a rather generous use of that term. Sure, there's the requisite red bridge, bamboo, and ponds. But what the garden lacks in orderliness it makes up for in charm—a hodgepodge of hedges whose roots go back to 1956, when it began as a generic garden.

Exit the Japanese Garden by climbing the short staircase tucked behind a waterfall. It will take you to another diamond in the rough—the Heroes Golf Course. This is a nifty, inexpensive nine-hole course that is also run by veterans and open to the public. Odds are good that you'll find a chatty worker inside its chalk-green Quonset hut clubhouse who's eager to share the story behind its American flag made entirely out of colored golf tees . . . or any other topic.

> **PICNIC OP**
>
> Next to the Japanese Garden are a dozen picnic tables that front a stage, where the Shakespeare Center of Los Angeles performs plays during the summer.

Leave the golf course by retracing your steps along Patton, which turns into Bonsall. Stay on Bonsall past the Brentwood Theatre—a movie and entertainment facility built in 1942, now privately owned—**until Bonsall becomes Vandergrift Avenue. Take Vandergrift until you hit Bonsall again, and turn right. Follow Bonsall for two blocks, then go right on Pershing Avenue. One block**

later, turn left on Dewey Avenue. Coming up on your right, you'll see an unhitched trailer splashed in star-spangled red, white, and blue . . . and camouflage. Behold the Freedom Barber Shop, also open to the public. The trailer's tongue-in-cheek decor (one sign declares, "No Smoking. Explosive Ammunition") tells you everything you need to know about its owner. Known for his bad jokes but big heart, "Dreamer" will often make house calls to vets who are bed-bound. Those who can't afford a cut are allowed to barter, accounting for the assortment of bric-a-brac inside.

Turn left on Grant Avenue, then right on Bonsall. As you approach Wilshire Boulevard, you'll come to a decrepit Victorian chapel on your right. Built in 1900, the Historic-Cultural Monument is recognized as the oldest building on Wilshire. Just past the chapel, Bonsall goes under Wilshire. The bridge is decorated inside and out by veterans, each mural telling a different story of American heroism.

Stay on Bonsall until you reach the T-intersection in front of the VA Hospital, then turn right on Dowlen Drive. After curving around for 1,200 steps, turn left on the street that heads toward the VA Hospital. Once the street ends, continue on the picturesque walkway that skirts the west end of the hospital and lets you back out to the T-intersection. Return to the National Cemetery by taking Bonsall north, then hang a right on Constitution. Follow Constitution under the freeway, across Sepulveda, and back to your car.

Driving home, you're suddenly struck with an odd appreciation for the privilege of braving Westside traffic.

43

CULVER CITY

GOODBYE, YELLOW BRICK ROAD

With apologies to West Hollywood, Culver City is the Southland's true Creative City. Random zoetropes, outrageous architecture, and more public art than you'll find in most museums—all are part of our journey into the heart of the original Oz.

■ **TERRAIN:** Flat
■ **SURFACE:** Paved
■ **FIDO FRIENDLY?:** Yes
■ **PARKING:** Street parking on Lucerne Avenue, near its junction with Duquesne Avenue, Culver City

L ike an old mining town whose fortunes exploded after the Gold Rush, Culver City once experienced a similar seismic shift. In 1920, a few years after its founding by Harry H. Culver, the town's population of 503 was still less than the number of people who puttered around Avalon on Catalina Island. Four years later, however, the opening of Metro-Goldwyn-Mayer Studios woke up the drowsy burg. Monumental classics like *The Wizard of Oz, Gone with the Wind, Singing in the Rain*, and *Ben-Hur* were filmed at the block-long studio and its satellite lots. By the 1940s, the "Heart of Screenland" was home to *half* of America's movie production, its borders swallowing up neighboring communities. This deep-rooted heritage of the arts and the byzantine layout brought about by incremental expansion have made Culver City what it is today.

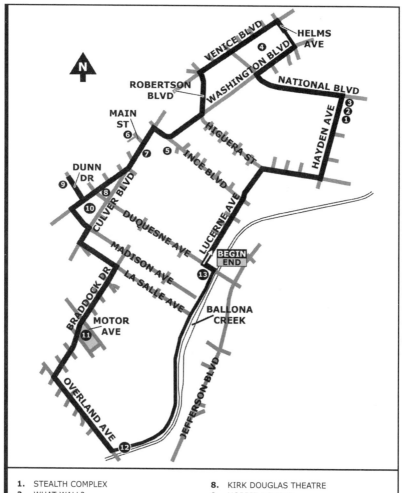

1. STEALTH COMPLEX
2. WHAT WALL?
3. SAMITAUR TOWER
4. HELMS BAKERY (FORMER LOCATION)
5. CULVER STUDIOS
6. ZOETROPE
7. CULVER HOTEL
8. KIRK DOUGLAS THEATRE
9. HOBBIT HOUSES
10. MGM STUDIOS (FORMER LOCATION)
11. DR. PAUL CARLSON PARK
12. BALLONA CREEK BIKE PATH
13. *RIVERS OF THE WORLD* MURAL

From its intersection with Duquesne Avenue, pro-ceed several blocks northeast on Lucerne Avenue. Turn right on Higuera Street, an orderly street of well-main-tained trees and homes that define the Culver City residential aesthetic. **Turn left on Hayden Avenue,** entering Hayden Tract, a once-forgotten industrial corner that has bloomed anew under the vision of architect Eric Owen Moss.

Over the next three blocks, you'll find some of the boldest contemporary buildings in the Southland. And certainly the oddest cactus garden. At 3585 Hayden, look behind the parking lot to your left. The cacti are affixed to a steel frame, suspended thirty-five feet in the air to maximize sun exposure. At 3528 is a complex known as the Stealth due to its resemblance to a stealth bomber. Its black, angular metal lies in stark contrast to the blocky concrete-and-wood structure across the street.

Just past the Stealth, note the 165-foot-long cement wall of the adjacent building. One-third of the way down is a protruding conference room. Its warped windows and shingled siding bust right through the flatness, as if to say, "What wall?" Reflecting Moss's wry parlance, that also happens to be the name of this wall.

Moss's crowning achievement, however, is the Samitaur Tower on the corner of Hayden and National Boulevard. All jutting forms, obtuse angles, and stacked steel rings, it looks like something a kid might throw together. Situated across from the Metro Expo line, the seventy-two-foot-tall monolith stands as a conspicuous testament to Culver City's creative energy while also proclaiming, "Dorothy, we're not in Kansas anymore." (Sorry, someone had to say it.)

By this point, you will have walked 2,000 steps. **Turn left on National, staying on the south side of the street. Turn right on Washington Boulevard, then left on Helms Avenue,** a pedestrian plaza that hosts outdoor summer movie nights. This is the Helms Bakery District, named after the former Helms Bakery to your left. The Art Deco compound was built in 1930 and was the official bakery for the 1932 Los Angeles Olympics. Its warehouses now house upscale furniture stores along Venice Boulevard.

Turn left on Venice, staying on the south sidewalk, then go left on Robertson Boulevard. It connects with Washington after one block. On the southwest corner of Washington and Ince Boulevard is a white colonial mansion that was used in the opening credits of *Gone with the Wind*. The historic Culver Studios was built by wunderkind producer Thomas H. Ince in 1919. He would die under mysterious circumstances at age forty-two just five years later.

Follow Washington as it swings northwest, then make a sharp left on Culver Boulevard. In one block, you'll come to Main Street, which extends all of about 400 feet. Its Lilliputian length is no accident. When he was designing his city, Harry Culver wanted a marketing hook, so he created what he claimed was "the shortest Main Street in America." Who can resist such pointless boosterism? Park yourself at one of Main Street's outdoor cafés and check off a new, unexpected item on your bucket list.

Main Street holds another surprise. **About 100 steps away from its junction with Culver, turn down the pedestrian alleyway to the left.** Notice the black, cylindrical object on a stand. This is a zoetrope, one of dozens clustered around Culver Boulevard that celebrate the city's cinematic legacy. Rotate the zoetrope's drum and peer through its slits, paying attention to the images inside the drum. Thanks to the "persistence of vision" phenomenon, the figures blend together to create a seamless moving image. A map to other zoetropes is displayed nearby, creating a fun scavenger hunt for another day.

EXTRA STEPS

Continue to the end of Main Street to reach what many consider the quirkiest collection of curios in Los Angeles—the Museum of Jurassic Technology, at 9341 Venice Boulevard. If you visit, find your way to the little-known rooftop garden and aviary, where tame birds serenade you while eyeing the butter cookie you just snagged from the museum's Russian Tea Room.

Double back on Main Street and note the triangular brick building on the southwest corner of Culver and Main. The 1924 Culver Hotel is a recognized historic landmark in more ways than one. All 124 Munchkins from *The Wizard of Oz* stayed here while filming at nearby MGM Studios. Duck inside its bar, which recreates a 1920s speakeasy. Its signature drink: the Red Slipper. Photos both inside and outside the hotel truly make Culver City's past come alive. On your way out, have a seat next to Harry Culver himself. His bronze likeness is reading a newspaper on a park bench. Check out the article he's reading for an amusing "meta" moment.

Head one block west of the hotel, where Culver reunites with Washington. Here you'll find the Washington Building, another triangular gem from the '20s. **Cross over to the north side of Washington,** which provides a nice view of the building's colonnade.

At the end of the block is the Kirk Douglas Theatre. Once known as the Culver Theatre, it has since been converted to a playhouse while still preserving its original Streamline Moderne elements and Culver neon sign.

One block past the theater, turn right on Dunn Drive. Toward the end of the block on the left, you'll come across a cottage that looks like a giant mushroom. This Historic-Cultural Monument is one of several storybook structures here, all designed by Lawrence Joseph, a former Walt Disney artist. The cottages are known as "the Hobbit Houses." What is it about Culver City and fictitious little people?

Turn around and continue west on Washington. Across the street, Sony Pictures sits in the footprint of the old Metro-Goldwyn-Mayer Studios, where the Yellow Brick Road and Hollywood's greatest musicals came to life. The studio actually covered six separate lots, spilling across Overland Avenue to the west and Jefferson Boulevard to the south. MGM's decline began after World War II, and by the 1960s, the "city within a city" had started selling off its assets to real-estate developers, much as 20th Century Fox did when its backlot became Century City.

Go left on Madison Avenue, right on Culver, and left on La Salle Avenue, re-entering Culver City's residential district. From La Salle, turn right on Braddock Drive, walk- ing **1,000 paces until you get to Overland. Hang a left, staying on the eastern sidewalk. After 800 steps, you'll come to an opening on the left with a blue sign marking the entrance to the Ballona Creek Bike Path.**

Head through the gates and continue along the pathway for about 1,000 steps, exiting at Duquesne. As you approach that street, look across the river for the metallic structure that appears to be a giant hand grenade but is actually a representation of a water urn. It was designed by Don Merkt as an homage to La Ballona Creek and its importance to the Tongva Indians. For a last gasp of public art, behold the *Rivers of the World* mural on your left as you **exit the bike path.**

After making a left on Duquesne, it's a short trek to your car. Your adventure through Screenland is now complete.

STEPPING BACK

Many of the residential blocks north and south of here rose from the ashes of MGM's studio lot. How can you tell which ones? Easy. Glance at a map for streets named after MGM's biggest stars—Astaire Avenue, Garland Drive, Lamarr Avenue, and Fairbanks Way and Pickford Way (side by side, of course).

PICNIC OP

Dr. Paul Carlson Park, 10400 Braddock Drive, where it intersects with Motor Avenue.

44

FRANKLIN CANYON

THE CENTER OF IT ALL

Many of us act like we're the center of the universe, but only Franklin Canyon can boast about being the true center of Los Angeles. Find out how in this rustic roundabout past the world's most famous fictional fishing hole.

- ■ **TERRAIN:** Flat with moderate inclines and one steep, short incline
- ■ **SURFACE:** Paved and unpaved
- ■ **FIDO FRIENDLY?:** Yes
- ■ **PARKING:** Lot at Coldwater Canyon Park and TreePeople, 12601 Mulholland Drive, Los Angeles

One of the great things about living in Los Angeles is our proximity to nature. Seventeen million people live within one hour of the Santa Monica Mountains, which extend from Griffith Park to Oxnard. In fact, L.A. is the only major city in the world divided by a mountain range. I was fortunate to have grown up in a house where the Santa Monicas were literally my backyard, leading to many safaris through the sumac. Thanks to the Santa Monica Mountains Conservancy, over 72,000 acres of parkland remain preserved, many of them in highly dense areas like the one wedged between Beverly Hills and Studio City.

Begin your walk in the parking lot for TreePeople, whose name sounds like a long-lost Sid & Marty Krofft project but is actually a nonprofit organization. Located on the grounds of an old fire station, it sprang from the teenage brain

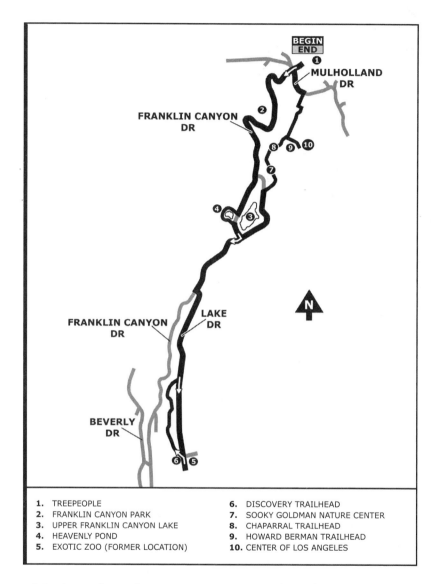

1. TREEPEOPLE	6. DISCOVERY TRAILHEAD
2. FRANKLIN CANYON PARK	7. SOOKY GOLDMAN NATURE CENTER
3. UPPER FRANKLIN CANYON LAKE	8. CHAPARRAL TRAILHEAD
4. HEAVENLY POND	9. HOWARD BERMAN TRAILHEAD
5. EXOTIC ZOO (FORMER LOCATION)	10. CENTER OF LOS ANGELES

of Andy Lipkis, who in 1974 was inspired to plant smog-tolerant trees throughout Los Angeles. I was one of Andy's first "volunteers" (forced by Mom during a scorching summer, thus the air-quotes) to help plant seedlings in soil-filled milk cartons for transport.

The TreePeople grounds have come a long way since then.

Take a moment to visit its learning center and gardens, which are nourished by a giant underground cistern. The center also serves as a starting point for a series of trails that extend as far east as Laurel Canyon.

Exiting the parking lot, cross the funky intersection to access Franklin Canyon Drive, which eventually connects with Beverly Drive to the south. After a few hundred feet, the mountain lane leaves a residential area and plunges into quiet wilderness. Hard to believe you're only ten minutes from the Beverly Hills Hotel. **Following a hairpin turn, the road dips into a canopy of trees—the entrance to Franklin Canyon Park.**

After passing a stop sign, bear right, staying on Franklin Canyon Drive. You are now on a perimeter road that loops around the three-acre Upper Franklin Canyon Lake, which comes into view on your left. The lake began as a reservoir in 1914, one of several built by William Mulholland to store water from the Los Angeles Aqueduct. It was taken

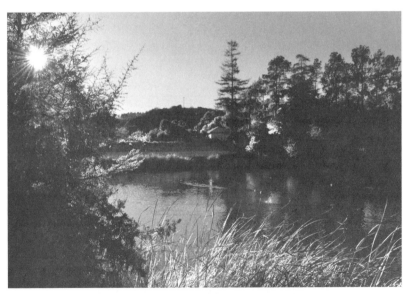

Upper Franklin Canyon Lake is a true gem of the Santa Monica Mountains.

offline after the 1971 Sylmar Earthquake. Its secluded yet convenient location has long made it a favorite for Hollywood studios filming everything from Oscar winners (*It Happened One Night, Silence of the Lambs, Platoon*) to, well, non-Oscar winners (*Big Momma's House, A Nightmare on Elm Street, Creature from the Black Lagoon*). Most famously, it's where Andy and Opie go fishing in the opening credits of *The Andy Griffith Show*, accompanied by that catchy whistling that has now just wormed its way into your brain (sorry).

Two thousand steps into your walk, turn right at the sign for Heavenly Pond and stroll around its tranquil waters, featured in the 1981 movie *On Golden Pond*. Keep an eye out for turtles clambering onto low-lying tree branches, often stacked up in little turtle pyramids.

> **PICNIC OP**
>
> Find a picnic table at the far end of Heavenly Pond, or a table under the redwoods that line the western shoreline of Upper Franklin Canyon Lake.

After looping around the pond, continue south on Franklin Canyon Drive. The road goes over a small dam, affording an excellent view of the lake. **Past the dam, turn right and follow the road downhill.** After 600 steps, you'll come to an old red-tiled abode at the intersection of Franklin Canyon and Lake Drive. **Turn left on Lake,** a pleasant and flat straightaway through a glen that extends to the southern portion of Franklin Canyon Park.

Lake ends 1,600 steps later at a closed gate with LADWP signs. Beyond the gates is the Lower Franklin Canyon Reservoir, off-limits to the public. **This is your turn-around point. Head north,** noticing the large grass field to your right. When I was a kid, we used to drive by to see the llamas in this field, part of an exotic zoo kept by a family who lived in the Spanish-style ranch house. It was built by oil baron Edward Doheny as a summer retreat. He preferred cattle.

Just past the drive-
way that leads to the
house—and just *be-*
fore **the driveway for**
a public parking lot—

SIDE-STEP

If you prefer not to take Discovery
Trail—sparing yourself a few burs in
your socks—just stay on Lake Drive.

find the trailhead on the left side of the road. Discovery Trail winds through chaparral and native trees like
oak and California black walnut. It parallels Lake Drive for 600
steps before rejoining the road.

Continue up Lake until it merges with Franklin Can-
yon Drive. Take this street back to the dam, only this
time continue straight ahead, hugging the eastern por-
tion of Upper Franklin Canyon Lake. The small wall separating the road from the lake is another WPA job. Feel free to
to veer off and meander through the cattails along the shoreline before linking up again with the main road.

Once the reservoir recedes from view, look for a
driveway on the right side. It leads to the Sooky Goldman
Nature Center, named after a vigilant conservationist who
helped protect Franklin Canyon from development. Take a
breather in the air-conditioned mini-museum, exploring its
hands-on exhibits. If you've seen any wildlife on your trip,
be sure to tell the volunteers. They'll put it on their "wildlife
sightings" whiteboard, which, the last time I was there, included a raccoon family, several quail, a red-tailed hawk, and a
bobcat (although there were some who swore it was a juvenile
mountain lion).

Leaving the nature center, head down the western
walkway to the dirt parking lot and turn right. At the
end of the lot, climb over the dirt berm marking the
trailhead for Chaparral Trail, a wide firebreak that of-
fers a shortcut back to your car. Before you climb its 400-
step ridgeline, however, one more prize awaits.

Just to the right of the trail—100 steps from the
trailhead—look for a clearing. Find the sign that says

"Howard Berman Trail" and railroad ties forming little steps in the dirt. To the left of the steps, under an oak tree, is a plaque set in concrete that includes latitude and longitude figures. As everyone knows, Los Angeles's boundaries are jagged and asymmetrical. But according to the National Park Service, this very spot provides order to the chaos, for it is the *exact geographic center* of Los Angeles. By extension, doesn't that mean that, at this very moment, *you're* the exact center of the L.A. universe, too? Don't let it go to your head . . .

Now that you've recalibrated your inner compass, **rejoin the trail and take it up the hill to the parking lot for Fire Station #108 at 12520 Mulholland Drive. Exit the lot and turn left on Mulholland, then walk one block to get back to TreePeople, on your right-hand side.**

45

BEVERLY HILLS

9021-*OH-OH!*

It's free to walk through one of the nation's richest zip codes, but living here will cost you an arm and a leg . . . sometimes, worse. You can always stay at its landmark hotel but just remember: you can check in, but you can't check out.

- ■ **TERRAIN:** Flat with stairs, gradual inclines, and one steep, short incline
- ■ **SURFACE:** Mostly paved
- ■ **FIDO FRIENDLY?:** No (not allowed at Greystone Park and Mansion)
- ■ **PARKING:** Lot at 485 Rodeo Drive, Beverly Hills

Like so much of Southern California's narrative, Beverly Hills' origins are a mix of oil and water. In the early 1900s, prospector Burton E. Green struck out trying to find black gold in the region. But he did stumble on a huge water table, forming the Rodeo Land and Water Company. He then subdivided the land and renamed it "Beverly Hills" after Beverly Farms in his native Massachusetts. From those humble beginnings came the 90210 area code, where, as Mr. Burton learned over a century ago, what lies beneath the surface is not always what you suspect.

From Santa Monica Boulevard, head north on Rodeo Drive. Your first destination is a domicile at 507 Rodeo that looks like a wedding cake. **Tread a few steps west on Park Way** to view the house and really appreciate its white-frosting flourishes that recall the architectural style of Antonio Gaudi.

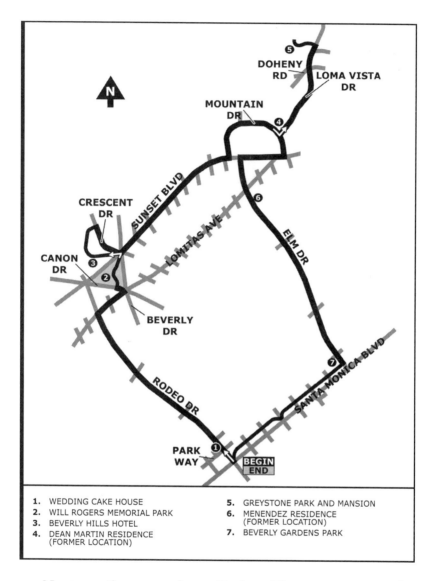

1. WEDDING CAKE HOUSE
2. WILL ROGERS MEMORIAL PARK
3. BEVERLY HILLS HOTEL
4. DEAN MARTIN RESIDENCE (FORMER LOCATION)
5. GREYSTONE PARK AND MANSION
6. MENENDEZ RESIDENCE (FORMER LOCATION)
7. BEVERLY GARDENS PARK

Next, **continue north on Rodeo.** The grass strip in the middle of the street used to be an equestrian trail known as "Ye Bridle Path" that led to hillside homes north of Sunset Boulevard. **Turn right on Lomitas Avenue.** After 200 steps, you'll come to a massive intersection with a six-way stop. On your left, bisected by Canon and Beverly Drives, you'll see Will

Rogers Memorial Park, named after the entertainer who was Beverly Hills' first honorary mayor.

Access the six-step staircase that leads to the gardens. When the Beverly Hills Hotel opened in 1912 across the street—back when Sunset was still a country lane—this park functioned as the entrance to the hotel. Sadly, it took George Michael to really put the park on the map. The pop singer was busted by an undercover cop for lewd acts in its restroom.

Cross Sunset where it intersects Crescent

STEPPING BACK

A pedestrian tunnel used to exist here, starting just to the left of the park's short staircase (look for the indentation where a palm is growing). It passed under Sunset and led to the hotel's lobby. As a kid, I became obsessed with getting into that old tunnel. Back then, its entrance was boarded up with an ill-fitting green door, its cracks just wide enough for my flashlight beam to penetrate the dark cobwebby passageway as I searched in vain for mummified bodies.

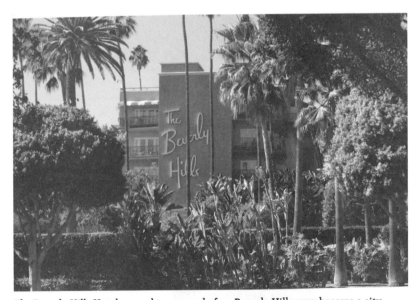

The Beverly Hills Hotel opened two years before Beverly Hills even became a city.

**and Beverly Drives. Proceed up Crescent, s?
left side.** On your left you'll see the iconic Beverly Hill.
tel, whose signature façade and grand bell towers grace the
cover of the Eagles' *Hotel California* album. Enter the famous
banana-leaf-wallpapered lobby via the hotel's long driveway.
Everyone who was anyone has patronized the "Pink Palace."
Frank Sinatra's Rat Pack used to hold court in its Polo Lounge,
which has arguably seen more A-list celebrities than any eatery in the world. If you subscribe to the "you only live once"
school of thought, book ahead for a reservation. Otherwise, sidle up to the luncheon counter in the Fountain Coffee Room,
which has been serving up comfort fare like frothy milkshakes
(beloved by Marilyn Monroe) and grilled cheese sandwiches
since 1949.

Vacate the lobby through its northern doors, following
signs to the hotel's famed bungalows. Elizabeth Taylor had
six of her eight honeymoons here. Other celebrities, drawn
by the bungalows' privacy and spaciousness, used them as
extended-stay homes. Howard Hughes rented out Bungalow
4 for years. He had the staff leave roast beef sandwiches in a
tree outside. Of course, it was this same seclusion that led to
the bungalows' reputation as an asylum for sexual peccadillos.

**Leaving the hotel grounds, return to Sunset and turn
left, staying on the north sidewalk.** As with the median on
Rodeo Drive, Sunset's used to be a bridle trail where the likes
of Mary Pickford and Douglas Fairbanks once cantered up to
the hotel from their nearby estate.

**Stay on Sunset for 1,800 paces. When you get to
Mountain Drive, make a left. Follow the street to 601,**
which used to be Dean Martin's pad.

Turn left at the corner of Loma Vista Drive. At 800
steps, you'll find the entrance to Greystone Park and Mansion. Push up the long driveway—a short but steep climb—
and explore the sumptuous eighteen-acre domain. The
46,000-square-foot manor (tours by appointment only) was

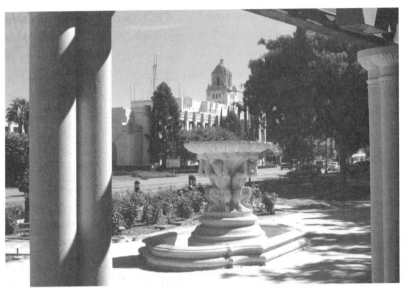

Ornate flourishes mark Beverly Gardens Park and Beverly Hills City Hall, both built in the early 1930s.

completed in 1928 for the son of oil tycoon Ed Doheny, the inspiration for the movie *There Will Be Blood*. But son Ned didn't have much time to enjoy it. In 1929, he was gunned down in the middle of the night by a disgruntled business associate, who then turned the gun on himself. The motive behind the murder-suicide remains unclear to this day.

Exit Greystone and head south on Loma Vista, then turn left on Mountain. Crossing Sunset, walk three blocks west and make a left on Elm Drive. At 722 Elm is another house that was rocked by tragedy. This is where the Menendez brothers killed their wealthy parents in cold blood in 1989 as they were watching TV, then went on a $1 million shopping spree. They are currently serving life without parole.

Continue south to Santa Monica Boule-

> **PICNIC OP**
>
> Find a shady bench along Beverly Gardens Park, which runs alongside Santa Monica Boulevard.

vard. Just before you get to the stop sign for that street, turn right on the dirt walkway of Beverly Gardens Park, which runs the length of Beverly Hills from Doheny to Whittier Drives. Keep an eye out for the landmark Beverly Hills sign and restored lily pond between Canon and Beverly.

    One block past Beverly, return to your car at Rodeo and Santa Monica . . . if not richer, then at least a little bit wiser.

46

BEVERLY HILLS II

ABOVE AND BELOW THE TRACKS

This 90210 tour is a two-parter. The first half homes in on lifestyles of the rich and famous. The second half is strictly business, zigzagging through the city's vaunted Golden Triangle.

- **TERRAIN:** Flat with gradual inclines
- **SURFACE:** Mostly paved
- **FIDO FRIENDLY?:** Yes
- **PARKING:** Lot at 485 Rodeo Drive, Beverly Hills

Up until the 1970s, residents of Beverly Hills were commonly lumped into two categories: "above the tracks" and "below the tracks." The "tracks" were in fact a Southern Pacific railway that ran alongside Santa Monica Boulevard, dividing that street into its familiar nicknames of Big Santa Monica and Little Santa Monica. If you resided "below the tracks," it was assumed that you lived in an apartment, a working-class underbelly memorialized in the movie *Slums of Beverly Hills*. Of course, living "above the tracks" came with its own set of problems, as seen in the movie *Down and Out in Beverly Hills*, in which we learn that husbands sleep with maids and neighbors like Little Richard pop in at the most inopportune times to screech out tunes on the piano.

This walk starts at that line of demarcation, in the Rodeo Drive parking lot between both Santa Monica Boulevards. The lot is situated in the former train track corridor.

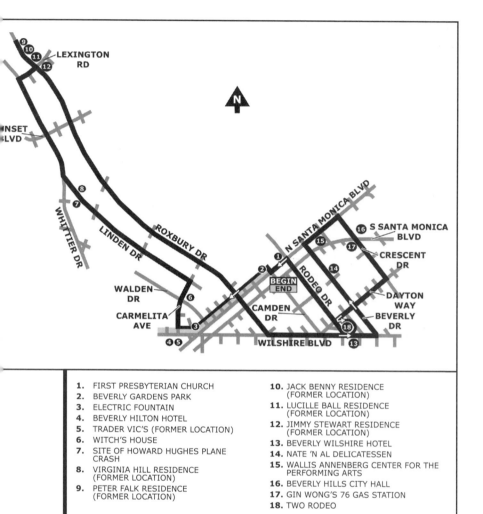

1. FIRST PRESBYTERIAN CHURCH
2. BEVERLY GARDENS PARK
3. ELECTRIC FOUNTAIN
4. BEVERLY HILTON HOTEL
5. TRADER VIC'S (FORMER LOCATION)
6. WITCH'S HOUSE
7. SITE OF HOWARD HUGHES PLANE CRASH
8. VIRGINIA HILL RESIDENCE (FORMER LOCATION)
9. PETER FALK RESIDENCE (FORMER LOCATION)
10. JACK BENNY RESIDENCE (FORMER LOCATION)
11. LUCILLE BALL RESIDENCE (FORMER LOCATION)
12. JIMMY STEWART RESIDENCE (FORMER LOCATION)
13. BEVERLY WILSHIRE HOTEL
14. NATE 'N AL DELICATESSEN
15. WALLIS ANNENBERG CENTER FOR THE PERFORMING ARTS
16. BEVERLY HILLS CITY HALL
17. GIN WONG'S 76 GAS STATION
18. TWO RODEO

Cross over to the northwest corner of Rodeo and Santa Monica. Jimmy Stewart's funeral was held at the nearly 100-year-old First Presbyterian Church here. It doubles as a preschool, where, as four-year-olds, my friends and I delighted in getting freight train engineers to blow their deafening horns as they rumbled past.

Continue west on Santa Monica. Once you pass Camden Drive, the sidewalk will turn into decomposed granite for much of the next five blocks. **Stroll through the Beverly Gardens Park green-**

PICNIC SPOT
Beverly Gardens Park, alongside Santa Monica Boulevard.

belt. After 800 steps, you'll reach the intersection of Santa Monica and Wilshire Boulevards. To your right you'll find the city's famous Electric Fountain, the first illuminated water display in the United States. It makes memorable cameos in the movie *Clueless* and the Go-Go's music video "Our Lips Are Sealed." Ruminate on the fountain's terra cotta tiles and relief carvings, which retrace California's history. The Native American woman praying for rain atop the fountain was created by the legendary sculptor Robert Merrell Gage.

Walk one block to the corner of Wilshire and Carmelita Avenue. Across the street is the famed Beverly Hilton Hotel. Notice the clumps of Tahiti-style palm trees lining the hotel's street-level façade, remnants of the tiki-mad Trader Vic's bar and restaurant that defined this corner for decades.

Turn right on Carmelita. On the southeast corner of Carmelita and Walden Drive is a storybook cottage known as the Witch's House. It was built in 1921 by Harry Oliver, a fanciful Hollywood art director who also designed the Tam O'Shanter restaurant and the Van De Kamp's windmill. Almost everything about its exterior is crooked or warped. Throw in its faded orange walls and it looks like a gingerbread house left out too long. Every Halloween in the '70s and '80s, the owner dressed as a witch and gave out Giant Taffy as she stirred her caldron of witch's brew (dry ice in water). Nowadays, under a new owner, Halloween trick-or-treaters sometimes flock here by the thousands!

From the Witch's House, head one more block east, then go left on Linden Drive. Though its residential portion only stretches a few blocks, Linden is ground zero for two horrific events involving two twentieth-century icons that happened within a year's time. On July 7, 1946, billionaire aviator Howard Hughes crashed an experimental airplane into a row of homes on Linden's 800 block. The residence at 805 sustained the worst damage when, according to the *Los Angeles Times*, "the plane's right wing sliced through the upstairs bedroom . . . narrowly missing the occupants." The plane ignited in a fireball, yet Hughes somehow survived the crash. The same can't be said about Bugsy Siegel, whose girlfriend Virginia Hill lived at 810 Linden. On the evening of June 20, 1947, the notorious gangster was reading a newspaper in Hill's living room when he was gunned down through a side window. The case was never solved.

Stay on Linden as it merges with Whittier Drive. Cross Sunset and make a right on Lexington Road. Stride one block to the intersection of Roxbury Drive. On the east side of the street are four consecutive homes known as Celebrity Row: 1004 Roxbury belonged to Peter Falk, 1002 to Jack Benny, 1000 to Lucille Ball, and 918 to Jimmy Stewart. Can you imagine the sort of block parties that must have gone on here?

From Jimmy Stewart's former house, it's 2,200 steps down Roxbury to Big Santa Monica. Continue another 400 paces, then go left onto Wilshire Boulevard. If you look at a map, you'll notice that you're slicing through the left corner of the so-called Golden Triangle, the retail-commercial core of the city and one of the most expensive parcels of real estate in the world. The triangle's base is formed by Wilshire, home to top talent agencies and Department Store Row—Neiman Marcus, Saks Fifth Avenue, and Barneys New York. Just past Barneys is the Beverly Wilshire Hotel, made famous as Julia Roberts's and Richard Gere's love nest in the movie *Pretty Woman*.

Turn left on Beverly Drive and head north. As you take in the street's boutiques, make sure to save room for lunch at Nate 'n Al Delicatessen at 414, a 1945 institution that is a second home for many Beverly Hills celebrities.

Turn right at Big Santa Monica, staying on the south sidewalk. On your immediate right you'll see the Wallis Annenberg Center for the Performing Arts. It was originally the Beverly Hills Post Office, a re-splendent Italian Renais-

> **STEPPING BACK**
>
> In general, Beverly Hills has a poor record when it comes to preserving historic structures. The city razed a number of grand movie palaces near Wilshire Boulevard, including the Art Deco-style Warner Beverly Hills, and the Beverly Theater, which had a Taj Mahal-type dome.

sance-style edifice from the 1930s whose echoey hallway leading to the auditorium has been nicely preserved.

Make a right on Crescent Drive, which forms the right side of the Golden Triangle. On your left is another Italian Renaissance gem—Beverly Hills City Hall—which doubled as the police station in *Beverly Hills Cop.* At the end of the block, on the southwest corner of Crescent and Little Santa Monica, is a 76 station—architecturally, the most famous gas station in the Southland. It was designed by Gin Wong, the same guy behind LAX's Theme Building. With its upward-swooping canopy and other playful motifs, it's a textbook example of Googie architecture.

From Crescent, make a right on Dayton Way and take it to Rodeo Drive, which bisects the Triangle. Turn left. Then, just before Wilshire, turn left again to access Two Rodeo, a European-style shopping center with a cobble-stone street.

Waltzing through Two Rodeo will bring you back to the corner of Rodeo and Dayton. From there, continue up Rodeo Drive, whose high-end shopping district is known the world over. Besides the usual window-shopping, car-gazing, and people-watching, be sure to look down on occasion. Mimicking Hollywood's Walk of Fame, Beverly Hills has created the Rodeo Drive Walk of Style. Every year, the city adds placards in the sidewalk venerating famous fashionis-

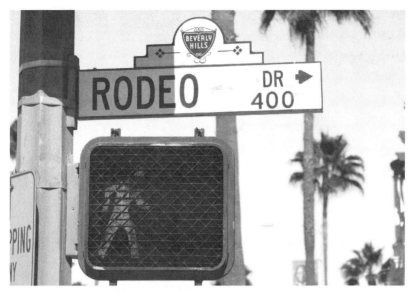

Walking is much easier on the wallet on Rodeo Drive.

tas, along with personal quotes. (Fred Hayman: "Clothes don't make a star. But they sure do help.")

Return to your car at Rodeo and Santa Monica in the "middle of the tracks," which, when all is said and done, is probably the best place to be.

Overleaf: The Manhattan Beach Pier.

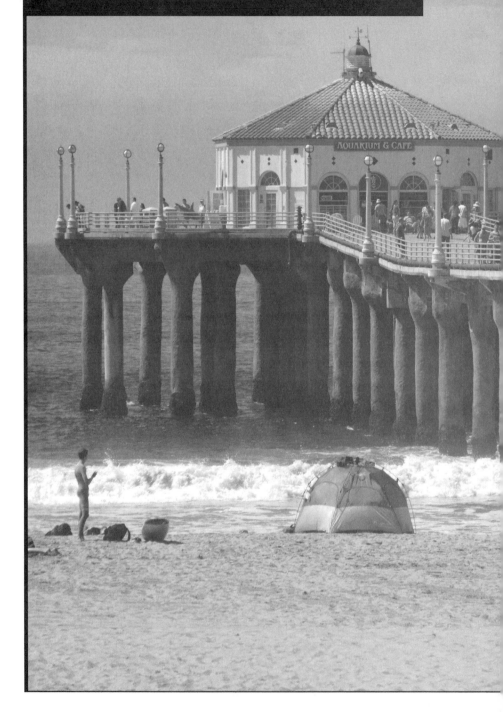

SOUTH BAY

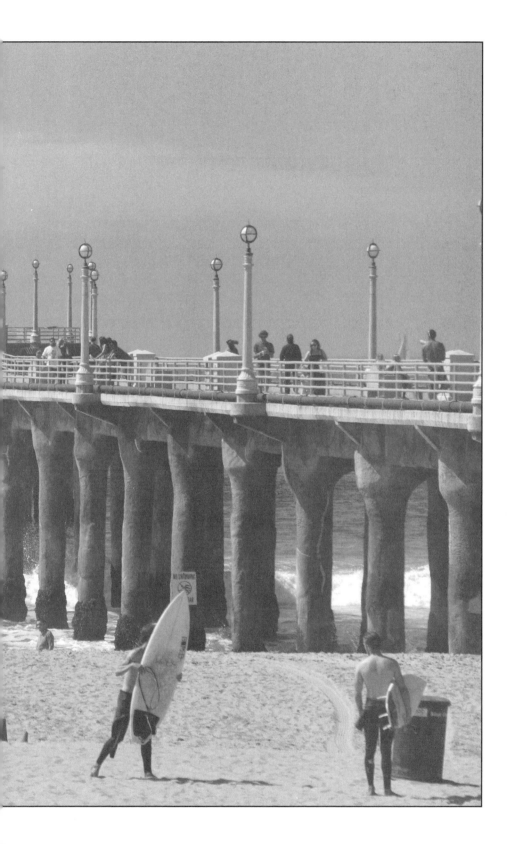

47

WESTCHESTER

MORE THAN JUST A PLANE VIEW

Westchester is home to the West Coast's busiest airport, but venture a little north and you'll find a sleepy vibe far removed from the bedlam, with an eye toward the ground to honor those who took to the skies.

- ■ **TERRAIN:** Flat
- ■ **SURFACE:** Mostly paved
- ■ **FIDO FRIENDLY?:** Yes
- ■ **PARKING:** Street parking on Sepulveda Westway, near its intersection with Westchester Parkway; lot at The Parking Spot, 9101 Sepulveda Boulevard, Los Angeles (proceed to the park directly south of The Parking Spot and In-N-Out Burger)

As picnic spots go, this one should be horrible. Sandwiched between a fast-food joint and two major boulevards, the feeble patch of grass on **the southwest corner of 92nd Street and Sepulveda Boulevard** offers no parking, no benches, and no amenities. But it does have one thing going for it that makes it truly one of the best places to picnic in L.A.—planes, and lots of them.

That's because this spot is directly under the flight path of incoming planes to Los Angeles International Airport. The presence of an In-N-Out Burger across the street only

PICNIC OP

The park at Sepulveda Boulevard and 92nd Street, across from In-N-Out Burger.

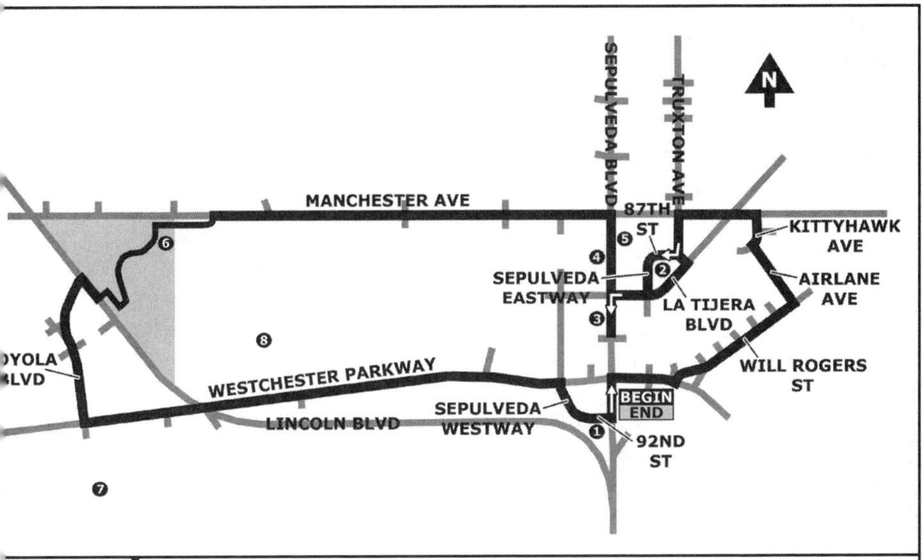

1. AIRPLANE-VIEWING GREENBELT
2. 87TH STREET TRIANGLE
3. AVIATION WALK OF FAME
4. MILLIRON'S DEPARTMENT STORE (FORMER LOCATION)
5. LOYOLA THEATER (FORMER LOCATION)
6. WESTCHESTER PARK
7. LAX
8. WESTCHESTER GOLF COURSE

adds to the unnamed park's allure. Get yourself a Double-Double (animal style, of course) and join the binocular-clad aviation enthusiasts on the grassy knoll. Thrill at the sight and sound of roaring passenger jets overhead, so close you can practically touch their hulking steel hulls as they gracefully touch down on the northern airstrip several hundred yards to the west.

From your runway rendezvous, head north one block to the intersection of Sepulveda and Westchester Parkway. Turn right on Westchester. After 200 steps, veer left at the fork onto Will Rogers Street. As its name suggests, you will suddenly find yourself in a wholesome residential district of well-tended gardens, Little League fields, and friendly neighbors working on boats. The rest of the streets are named after aviation terms or pioneers like Amelia Earhart.

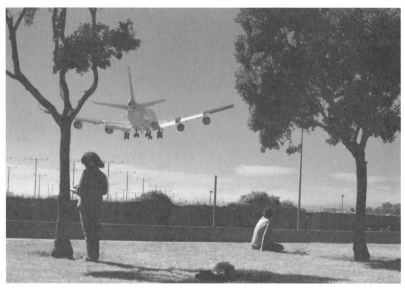

A big steel bird about to touch down on LAX's northern runway.

From Will Rogers, take Airlane Avenue up to Kittyhawk Avenue, then go right to Manchester Avenue. Walk two blocks west—past La Tijera Boulevard—and turn left at Truxton Avenue. After passing a nice restaurant, you'll come to the intersection of Truxton and 87th Street. This is the northeast point of a business district · called the 87th Street Triangle (an isosceles, if you want to get technical about it), a living throwback to the Westchester of yesteryear.

Indeed, many of these specialty shops have been around for decades, which explains the presence of a sewing shop, an "art shoppe," and a delightful independent record store with groovy '70s signage. To walk the triangle, which is very small, **go right on 87th Street till it bends southward toward La Tijera. Make a left on La Tijera, then another left on Truxton. When you hit 87th Street, you will have completed the triangle. Retrace your steps back to La Tijera and turn right. Upon reaching Sepulveda, cross over to**

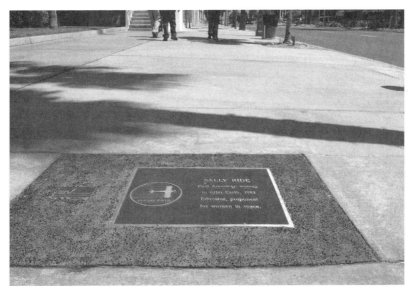

Astronaut Sally Ride gets a well-deserved plaque on the Aviation Walk of Fame.

the western sidewalk and turn left.

Just past the building on your right—the cornerstone of a shopping center—is a rotunda at the north end of the center's parking lot. The rotunda honors aeronautic and aerospace pioneers, and was commissioned by a nonprofit known as Flight Path. Taking a cue from Hollywood, Flight Path also created an Aviation Walk of Fame. There are at least a dozen plaques on the sidewalk and grass median between here and Howard B. Drollinger Way.

After acknowledging the winged heroes, **turn around and head north on Sepulveda, past La Tijera.** On your

EXTRA STEPS

There are several more plaques north and south of here on both sides of Sepulveda, including one extolling the male president of United Airlines who "made the 1930 decision to hire women to serve as flight attendants." Hmmm . . . you could argue that this decision made more of a contribution to men than it did to women.

immediate left is a discount department store housed in a huge mid-century building. It was designed by Holocaust survivor Victor Gruen, often credited as the inventor of the modern shopping mall. When Gruen opened Milliron's department store in 1949, it featured novel, car-friendly concepts like rooftop parking and display kiosks angled toward the street. Both features have since been stripped away (the kiosks have been replaced by palm trees fronting the brick walls). For decades, Milliron's—later changed to the Broadway department store—was the hub of a bustling corridor that also housed a Newberry's and a Woolworth, as well as soda fountains and a flagship movie theater, the Loyola. The defunct theater can be seen across the street at 8610 Sepulveda. Now a medical building, many of the features have been preserved, including the terrazzo sidewalk, the ticket window, and fluid lines that evoke waves and seashells. A swan still sits atop its sixty-foot-high tower.

At the next corner, link up again with Manchester. Turn left and stay on the south sidewalk. After 3,000 steps, you'll come across city tennis courts, part of a recreation center that includes a pool, gymnasium, and basketball courts. Find the walking trails into the park a few feet past the tennis courts. Amble through the park in a southwesterly direction until you come to Lincoln Boulevard. At its intersection with Loyola Boulevard, cross over to Loyola. Stay on the left side of the street, which has a wide walking lane. When you reach Westchester Parkway, cross the street and head east. Westchester Parkway eventually passes over Lincoln.

There's an urban legend that old tunnels run beneath the airport. That's partially true. Just south of here, engineers started to tunnel Lincoln under the north runways, but later scrapped the project. The tunnels still exist and are continually maintained for safety reasons . . . and to keep out the dreaded mole people.

After crossing Lincoln, Westchester Parkway becomes a pleasant but desolate thoroughfare, blazing a trail over the graves of hundreds of homes that were condemned during the LAX expansion in the 1960s. In all, 4,500 houses were torn down, and future airport development is not out of the question. Another casualty of the expansion was the Westchester Golf Course, visible to your left. Once an eighteen-hole golf course, it had three holes amputated, rendering it a fifteen-hole course. To keep things interesting, how great would it have been to play the final three holes on a runway, creating the ultimate hazard in dodging jets? Speaking of which, the view to your right offers another prime vantage point to see them coming in for landings.

After passing La Tijera, it's time to put down your own landing gear as you approach Sepulveda Westway, your round-trip arrival right on time for an In-N-Out shake to go!

48

EL SEGUNDO

A LITTLE NOSTALGIA TRIP

When Standard Oil opened its second refinery here in 1911, the city was christened El Segundo—Spanish for "The Second." Since then, the coastal community has clung to its small-town roots, making this breezy walk second to none.

■ **TERRAIN:** Flat with slight inclines
■ **SURFACE:** Mostly paved
■ **FIDO FRIENDLY?:** Yes
■ **PARKING:** Street parking near Library Park, 111 Mariposa Avenue, El Segundo (proceed to the park's entrance on Main Street)

Many Angelenos only know El Segundo from the commercial zone they see along Imperial Highway, El Segundo Boulevard, or Sepulveda Boulevard—wide thoroughfares with predictable franchise restaurants, aerospace industry holdouts, and sterile office towers housing Fortune 500 companies.

El Segundo, nestled between LAX and Manhattan Beach, is indeed all of those things. But the residential district west of Sepulveda is an entirely different Westside story, remaining remarkably resilient to change. If you want to experience a slice of Americana right in your own backyard, bust out your chinos and PF Flyers and make for this beach-adjacent enclave.

Start your walk at Library Park, an inviting public green with a central gazebo that seems straight out of the

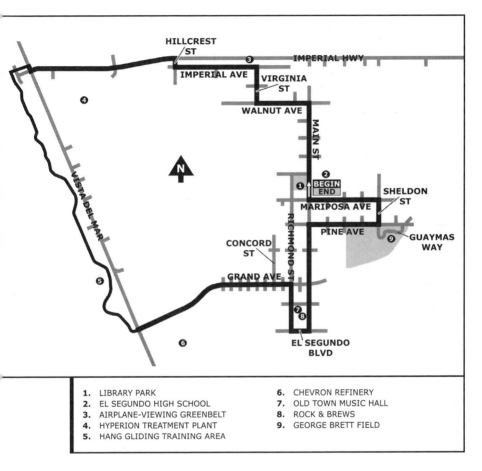

1. LIBRARY PARK
2. EL SEGUNDO HIGH SCHOOL
3. AIRPLANE-VIEWING GREENBELT
4. HYPERION TREATMENT PLANT
5. HANG GLIDING TRAINING AREA
6. CHEVRON REFINERY
7. OLD TOWN MUSIC HALL
8. ROCK & BREWS
9. GEORGE BRETT FIELD

1950s. During the summer, the park hosts popular summer concerts. Directly across the street is El Segundo High School, which claims to have appeared in more films and TV shows than any other high school in the world. One look at its stately brick façade and you can see why. Built in 1927, it has a timeless quality that fits our mental picture of what every campus should look like. Turns out, the school is one of beauty *and* brains. A 2008 study by a national magazine placed it in the top five percent of public schools in the country.

Continuing north on Main Street, you'll pass tree-oriented street names that evoke instant nostalgia—Oak, Maple,

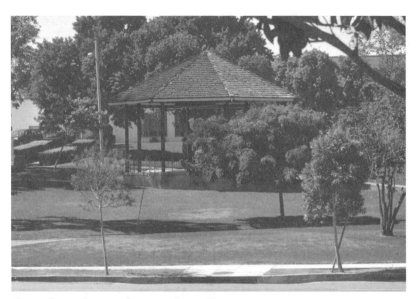

The gazebo at Library Park is a popular wedding spot.

Sycamore, Walnut. Despite the promises of their signs, I have yet to find any street lined with these trees. Regardless, the streets west of Main are awash with one-story homes with picket fences and wind chimes. **I recommend taking Walnut Avenue (three blocks north of the school),** which makes up for its lack of walnut trees with plenty of shade.

After a couple of blocks west on Walnut, turn right on Virginia Street. Take it for two blocks until you reach the T-intersection at Imperial Avenue. Cross the street to the greenbelt on a bluff, which offers a sublime view of the LAX runways across Imperial Highway.

Stay on the green-

EXTRA STEPS

Come Christmastime, no neighborhood in SoCal gets more decked out than the 1200 block of Acacia Avenue, otherwise known as Candy Cane Lane. Santa and his sleigh have been known to drop in. From Main Street, walk 1,200 steps east on Imperial Avenue, then turn right on Center Street. Acacia Avenue will be your left.

belt for two westward blocks until Imperial Avenue intersects with Hillcrest Street. As Hillcrest veers off to the left, find the pedestrian-only sidewalk on the right. Access this sidewalk to connect with Imperial Highway, a forty-one-mile road that predates the freeways and used to be the major connector between El Segundo and Anaheim.

Walking on the south sidewalk, head west on Imperial toward the beach. After one block, you'll notice a mysterious-looking compound behind barbed wire to your left. This is the Hyperion Treatment Plant—the oldest and biggest waste water facility in L.A., capable of treating almost a billion gallons of our ickiest matter per day! The plant doubled as the factory where wafers were manufactured in that schlock classic, *Soylent Green.* So perhaps its waste is not really waste. Perhaps . . . *it's people!*

Time to get your mind out of the sewer and back on the walk. **Cross over to the north side of Imperial Highway and use the crosswalk to get to the beach side of Vista Del Mar. A parking lot will appear before you. Stay on the sidewalk that parallels the lot's driveway. Continue on the dirt path that cuts through the ice plant and leads to the Dockweiler Bike and Pedestrian Path. Turn left and follow the trail along the beach.**

At the path's 1,000-step mark, notice the candy-cane-colored smoke stacks to your left, part of a fifty-five-acre plant owned by the Department of Water and Power that generates electricity. Its gas-powered steam turbines are cooled by seawater. In another 800 steps, just past a parking lot, you may come across a hang glider or two parked on the sand. Many hang gliding enthusiasts point to the coastal bluffs here as the site where the sport took off in 1966. Look for the placard paying tribute to this locale, an ideal spot for beginners with its "soft, gentle slopes and smooth coastal breezes."

Six hundred steps past the hang glider beach—just

beyond the beach volleyball courts—turn left at the end of a parking lot. Cross Vista Del Mar to the south side of Grand Avenue, which will return you to El Segundo.
As you walk up Grand, you will find yourself at the northwest corner of the 1,000-acre Chevron Refinery. Up through the 1920s, a long pier enabled boats to haul in crude oil, which the company refines to the tune of 290,000 barrels per day. Regardless of what one thinks about the burning of fossil fuels, El Segundo owes its existence to the petroleum giant, which built its tidy streets and supports its schools.

Continue east on Grand for 1,200 steps until you get to Concord Street. On the center median, you'll see a sign announcing that you are in downtown El Segundo, an enjoyably walkable stretch with a wealth of fine eating options. Despite the city's homespun feel, its restaurants have changed with the times . . . and tastes.

Two blocks later, make a right on Richmond Street. At 140 Richmond is the Old Town Music Hall, located in a nearly 100-year-old cinema. The cultural landmark shows silent movies accompanied by a massive 1925 Wurlitzer organ. The theater plays matinees on weekends, so if you plan your walk around their schedule, you'll be sitting pretty.

Continue on Richmond to the T-intersection of El Segundo Boulevard. Across the street is the employee entrance to the Chevron Refinery. Talk about a company town— up until the '50s, it was not uncommon for employees to be paid in scrip rather than dollars!

Proceed two blocks east and hang a left on Main. If you're a fan of good beer and music, stop in at Rock & Brews at 143 Main, co-owned by Paul Stanley and Gene Simmons from Kiss. Otherwise, keep walking on Main for three more blocks, which will bring you to more mom-and-pop businesses and restaurants.

Next, turn right on Pine Avenue. In two blocks you'll reach a park with baseball diamonds on your right. The field at

Pine and Guaymas Way, in the northeast corner, is George Brett Field. Brett is El Segundo's most fa-

PICNIC OP

Recreation Park at Pine Avenue and Guaymas Way.

mous son, a Hall of Fame baseball player drafted by the Kansas City Royals right out of El Segundo High in 1971. By the way, for those baseball fans out there, observe the tar-producing pine trees that encircle his dedicated baseball field. Think they're there to mock poor George?

From the park, head north on Sheldon Street, then left on Mariposa Avenue until it hits Library Park on Main. Time to make like Marty McFly and head back to the future.

49

MANHATTAN BEACH

PLEASANT STRAND, GNARLY SAND

More accessible than Santa Monica and less loopy than Venice Beach, Manhattan Beach offers all the familiar earmarks of a classic SoCal beach community. This circular route spotlights its most enchanting—and peculiar—features.

- ■ **TERRAIN:** Flat with slight inclines
- ■ **SURFACE:** Mostly paved
- ■ **FIDO FRIENDLY?:** Yes
- ■ **PARKING:** Street parking on Valley Drive, near its intersection with Elm Avenue, Manhattan Beach

O n the surface, Manhattan and Manhattan Beach couldn't be more different. But like the New York borough it's named after, this seaside city—incorporated in 1912—is marked by pricey real estate and an air of exclusivity. And yet, also like its East Coast namesake, it's highly walkable, with a vibrant outdoor culture and prevailing egalitarianism that keeps it from getting too pretentious.

From its intersection with Elm Avenue, cross over to the east side of Valley Drive to the wood-chip walking path, which cuts through a greenbelt known as Veterans

STEPPING BACK

Veterans Parkway was carved out of an old Santa Fe Railway right-of-way that was created in 1888. For almost 100 years, passenger and freight trains chugged through here, connecting Los Angeles to Redondo Beach.

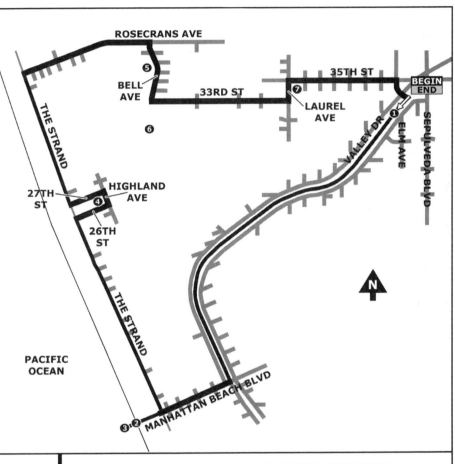

1. VETERANS PARKWAY
2. MANHATTAN BEACH PIER
3. ROUNDHOUSE MARINE STUDIES LAB AND AQUARIUM
4. BRUCE'S BEACH PARK
5. NATIONAL GUARD ARMORY
6. SAND DUNE PARK
7. TREE SECTION OF EAST MANHATTAN BEACH

Parkway. The trail runs along Valley all the way to Hermosa Beach, though you'll peel off after 2,600 steps. This is a winsome walk with cool ocean breezes and benches every quarter-mile. There are also drinking fountains for your canine companion. Note the prime real estate to the west of the parkway. Though the homes are small and close together, sale prices regularly start in the lower seven digits. Several of the streets have ornate gas street lamps.

Make a right when you reach Manhattan Beach Boulevard, a busy street with lots of fresh, tasty fare and local flavor. **Follow it downhill until it runs into the Manhattan Beach Pier.** The 1920 historic landmark is the oldest standing concrete pier on the West Coast. It was also one of the first places to host surfers, who've been weaving in and out of its pilings since the 1940s. **Roam to the end of its nearly 1,000-foot deck.** The octagonal building is home to a fish joint and the Roundhouse Marine Studies Lab and

> **EXTRA STEPS**
>
> Wanna tack on another 10,000 steps? Walk the Veterans Parkway all the way to its southern end, muscling up at its fitness stations along the way. The greenbelt terminates at the Redondo Beach Pier. Return the way you came or take the Strand back up to Manhattan Beach Boulevard.

> **PICNIC OP**
>
> Next to the Manhattan Beach Pier, along The Strand.

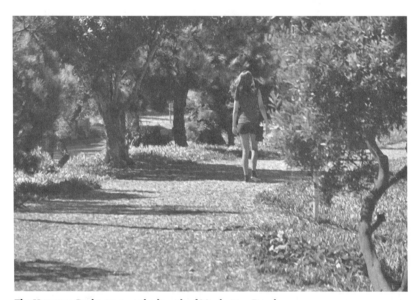

The Veterans Parkway runs the length of Manhattan Beach.

Aquarium. The aquarium (free, with suggested donations) is popular with school kids and features touch tanks, sharks, and other sea life.

Head back to the entrance of the pier, cross the bike path, and make a left on The Strand, following the pedestrian traffic up the coast. Manhattan Beach is popular with athletes, surfers, and young, upwardly mobile professionals. As such, you will notice more beautiful flesh per capita here than any other Southland beach. Fortunately, you are well-tuned to the art of covert ogling.

At The Strand's 1,400-step point—opposite a lifeguard station on the sand—access the walkway to your right. The walkway leads to 26th Street. Head up the gentle incline to Highland Avenue and go north. On your left, you'll find a small park that looms large in significance. Besides being the oldest park in Manhattan Beach, Bruce's Beach Park is a remnant of Bruce's Beach—once the only seaside resort in Los Angeles County that was open to all races and colors. As you walk north on Highland, don't miss the historical marker halfway down the block. It tells the story of the Bruces, an influential black couple who paved the way for minorities to settle in this part of town shortly after Manhattan Beach's founding.

Make a left on 27th Street and traipse back down to The Strand. Continue north until you get to Rosecrans Avenue. Head east on Rosecrans (admiring the surfboard-embedded artwork in its crosswalks) until you get to Bell Avenue. **Turn right on Bell.** On your right you'll find a National Guard armory, used since 1948 as a storage facility and training post. Just past the armory—at the corner of 33rd Street—you'll be greeted by a sign for Sand Dune Park. This may be the only city park in the country where you need to make a reservation to play in the sand.

Of course, it's not just any sand. With an elevation gain of 250 feet, the park's dune is more like a mountain. It has

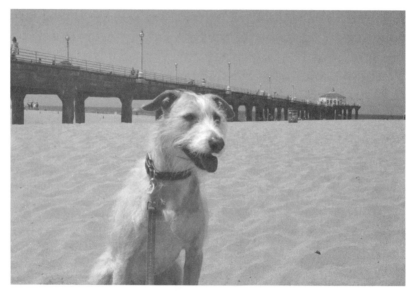

Even the dogs seem more beautiful at Manhattan Beach.

long drawn fitness buffs—everyone from regular folks to Kobe Bryant to the USC football team—who like to *feel the burn* by climbing its forty-five-degree slope. Concerned about wear and tear, the city implemented a reservation and fee system and divided the dune in half—the left side is for children, the right side for exercising adults. Children under thirteen and adults over fifty-five are exempt from reservations.

Leaving Sand Dune Park, proceed east on 33rd Street. Note the odd shoulders where people park their cars. They look like driveways but run parallel to the street, alternately surfaced by stone, brick, asphalt, concrete, or dirt. Are these private or public spaces?

Go left on Laurel Avenue. After one block, turn right on 35th Street. The next few blocks intersect several tree-named streets—part of the so-called Tree Section of East Manhattan Beach (the area closer to the beach is ingeniously known as the Sand Section). As with El Segundo, though, you won't find many of the trees that the streets are named after.

When you reach Elm Avenue, make a right and find your car. As you drive away, you resolve to reserve a spot on the city's website and tackle that monster dune for your next visit. And you'll do it *without* shoes, learning from a misguided author who emptied half the sand from Manhattan Beach onto his living room floor after he got home.

50

HERMOSA BEACH / REDONDO BEACH

PIER TO PIER

This easy out-and-back along the coast links Hermosa Beach with Redondo Beach and includes their very different piers. Added bonus: you're guaranteed to see whales . . . just not where you expect them to be.

- ■ **TERRAIN:** Flat with stairs
- ■ **SURFACE:** Paved
- ■ **FIDO FRIENDLY?:** Yes
- ■ **PARKING:** Lot on 11th Street, half a block west of Hermosa Avenue, Hermosa Beach

Though they're neighbors, about the only thing Hermosa Beach and Redondo Beach have in common is the beach. Hermosa draws a younger, rowdier crowd that betrays its legacy as a music and surfing mecca. Redondo Beach is more family- and boat-oriented, with a unique horseshoe-shaped pier full of colorful old salts. Much of this walk is on the promenade that links the two communities—part of a bike lane that, all told, runs twenty miles from Santa Monica to Redondo Beach.

From the parking lot at Hermosa Avenue and 11th Street, access the Hermosa Beach Pier by striding a few steps north on Hermosa before turning left on Pier Avenue, which is lined with raucous beach establishments. As you walk toward the pier, you'll notice some jazzy memorials in the plaza. No, seriously. Though L.A.'s Central Avenue may take issue, Hermosa Beach bills itself as "The Jazz Corner of the West." The tradition started in the late 1930s, when

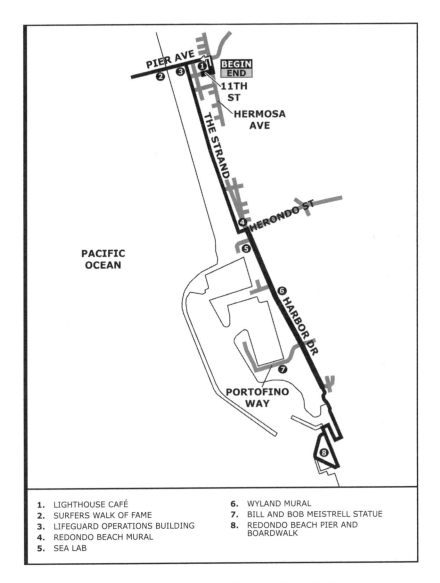

1. LIGHTHOUSE CAFÉ
2. SURFERS WALK OF FAME
3. LIFEGUARD OPERATIONS BUILDING
4. REDONDO BEACH MURAL
5. SEA LAB
6. WYLAND MURAL
7. BILL AND BOB MEISTRELL STATUE
8. REDONDO BEACH PIER AND BOARDWALK

hepcats congregated to places like the Hut Ballroom, a popular outdoor dance pavilion located right about where you're standing. The Lighthouse Café, to your left, has been hosting jazz concerts since 1949, ground zero for many famous live recordings. Pier Avenue contains several plaques on granite blocks honoring artists like Miles Davis and Dizzy Gillespie and dozens of others who played here.

Go a few steps west of the Lighthouse Café, where Pier Avenue turns into the Hermosa Beach Pier. The original wooden pier from 1904 was destroyed by storms, so up went the concrete fishing pier you see today. On your right, the bronze statue of a guy on a shortboard is that of Tim Kelly, a legendary surfer from the early '60s who also earned acclaim as a courageous lifeguard before he died at age twenty-four. In addition to honoring Kelly, a second plaque gives props to Hermosa Beach for its "a unique contribution . . . to professional lifesaving."

Halfway down the pier are even more tokens embedded in concrete. This is the Surfers Walk of Fame. One of the tablets credits Hermosa Beach as the original birthplace of surfing in California. If we've learned anything so far, it's that Hermosa isn't shy about laying claim to something. Farther south, Huntington Beach—aka, Surf City, USA—would beg to differ. So would Redondo Beach, which in 1907 hosted a

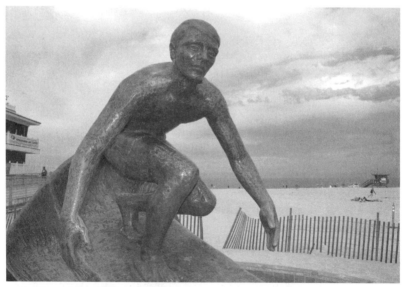

Surfing legend Tim Kelly eternally hangs ten at the entrance to the Hermosa Beach Pier.

surfing demonstration by pioneering surfer George Freeth, who gets his own plaque here. Not

> **PICNIC OP**
> Next to the Hermosa Beach Pier, along The Strand.

to be outdone, Redondo honors Freeth with a statue. But then, knowing how territorial surfers are, would you expect anything different from the cities where the sport came of age?

Walk to the end of the pier and enjoy the views. The Manhattan Beach Pier is visible to the north, while the southern sphere is dominated by the Palos Verdes Peninsula. **Turn around and head back to the pier's entrance. Just past the Lifeguard Operations building, turn right on The Strand**, following its stream of walkers and bicyclists. At its 1,400-step mark, The Strand makes a forty-five-degree left turn and enters Redondo Beach, reinforced by a long mural displaying the glories of Hermosa's southern neighbor. **The Strand ends at the corner of Herondo Street and Harbor Drive. Make a right on the sidewalk, heading south on Harbor.**

A block away is a street-level mural depicting sea life on the side of the SEA Lab, a little-known marine center that's open to the public and popular with schools. A few more steps to the right is a mosaic mural with beach-related imagery, part of the city's plan to beautify Harbor Drive. But the grand-daddy of Redondo's City Beautiful movement is just ahead at the generating plant, at 1100 Harbor. With the wall of the plant as his canvas, the artist Wyland created an 87-foot-tall, 622-foot-wide painting of migrating gray whales in the early '90s. The massive mural wraps around the southern wall. (Let Hermosa play the braggart; clearly Redondo is content with its public artwork.) Amazingly, Wyland freestyled the whole thing—no sketches, no preliminary outlines of the cetaceans. It's one of 100 "Whaling Wall" murals he created around the world. Enjoy this one while you can. The city's long-term goal is to tear this plant down and replace it with a mixed-use zone known as Harbor Village.

Three hundred steps past Portofino Way, Harbor veers off to the left at the stop sign. Do not follow it. Instead, continue straight on the sidewalk, which is joined by a bike path and enters a parking structure. A mural, natch, welcomes you to the Re-

> **EXTRA STEPS**
>
> Half a block past the whale mural, turn right on Portofino Way. On your left, 400 steps in, is a turnout for a seaside lagoon, where you'll find a statue of two sporting fellows. The brothers Bill and Bob Meistrell were identical twins who invented the modern wetsuit at their shop, Dive N' Surf, in the early 1950s. Though the brothers recently passed, the shop remains in business just a couple blocks away.

dondo Beach Pier and Boardwalk. At this point, you're homing in on the halfway point of our journey.

Drop down to the bottom portion (the boardwalk) and explore this historic pier. The pier's origins are over 100 years old. The first thing you'll notice is it's not a traditional

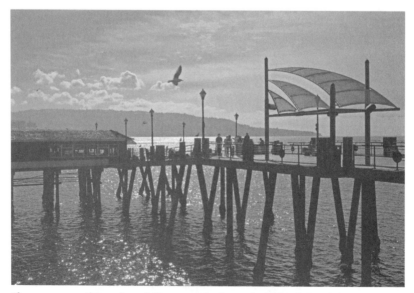

There are worse things than whiling away the day at the Redondo Beach Pier.

straight line extending into the surf; its current shape is the result of different wharfs that have virtually calcified together over the decades, making it the largest "endless" pier in California. The westernmost section loops out into the ocean like a backwards-sloping "D."

The pier's clientele reflects its willy-nilly layout. Diehard fishermen occupy the southern leg and newer, upscale restaurants jostle with shacky eateries and old arcades. Hands down, this pier has the most character of any in the Southland, and it will always have a special place in my eight-year-old heart. For it was here, during summer camp, where I caught my very first fish—a sand dab that I insisted my mother cook when we got home. It was rendered inedible by that time, so we fed it to a neighborhood cat.

After sampling some pier grub (you may even find sand dabs on the menu), **return to Hermosa Beach via the way you came.**

51

RANCHO PALOS VERDES

WALKING IN THE BLUFF

Orky and Corky are long gone, but Palos Verdes still offers thrills of a different sort—like this exhilarating out-and-back walk, high above the crashing Pacific that will make you feel like you're on top of the world.

- **TERRAIN:** Flat with slight inclines
- **SURFACE:** Paved and unpaved
- **FIDO FRIENDLY?:** Yes
- **PARKING:** Lot off of Calle Entradero, 0.2 miles west of Palos Verdes Drive W., Rancho Palos Verdes

Is there a more breathtaking stretch of coastline than the Palos Verdes Peninsula? Tongva Indians, Portuguese whalers, Japanese farmers, Mexican ranchers—just about everybody has had their piece of Palos Verdes pie, but it took a New York developer to buy out the store.

In 1913, Frank A. Vanderlip began to subdivide the 16,000-acre peninsula with the idea of making it "the most fashionable and exclusive residential colony" in America. But if there was a caveat emptor in his grand designs, it was the peninsula's notoriously brittle cliffs, which have led to several landslides over the years. The upside for us? Undeveloped seaside bluffs with unimpeded views of the ocean.

After parking your car in the Calle Entradero lot, walk to the southern end of the lot and access Golden Cove Trail. The pathway—well-marked with signs—is part of a 7.5-mile route some 185 feet above the Pacific through Vicente Bluffs Reserve. The bluffs are named after a former friar,

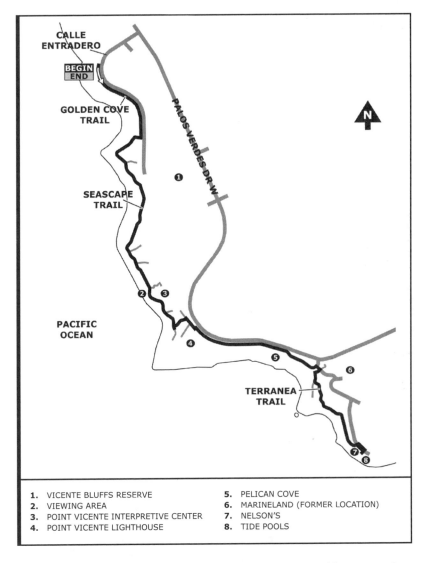

1. VICENTE BLUFFS RESERVE
2. VIEWING AREA
3. POINT VICENTE INTERPRETIVE CENTER
4. POINT VICENTE LIGHTHOUSE
5. PELICAN COVE
6. MARINELAND (FORMER LOCATION)
7. NELSON'S
8. TIDE POOLS

Vincente Santa Maria, from the old rancho era (the "n" in his name was eventually dropped).

The trail parallels Calle Entradero for the first 600 steps, at which point it veers right, descending toward the cliffs. Continue on this portion, known as Seascape Trail. Watch pelicans dive-bomb into the surf, and keep an eye out for the rare, inch-wide El Segundo blue butterfly, usually found on the bulbs of buck-wheat plants.

PICNIC OP
The stepped-concrete viewing area outside the Vicente Interpretive Center, 31501 Palos Verdes Drive W., facing the ocean.

In another 1,400 steps, you'll come across an amphitheater-type viewing area facing the ocean. This is a popular spot to watch for Pacific gray whales during their 12,000-mile migrations from Alaska to Baja California and back—thought to be the longest migration of any mammal on earth. The best time to spot them is in November and December, and again in March and April. Even if the whales fail to put on a show, you still stand a good chance of witnessing frolicking dolphins.

From the viewing area, head up the pathway to the front entrance of the Point Vicente Interpretive Center, marked by a breaching gray whale sculpture. Up until the 1980s, this was a firing range used by the military. As the

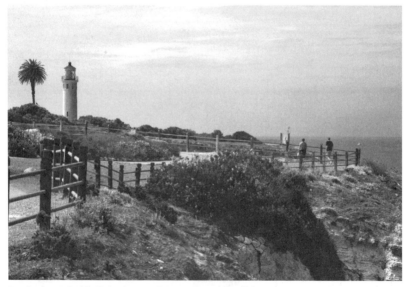

Trails along the bluffs lead toward Point Vicente Lighthouse.

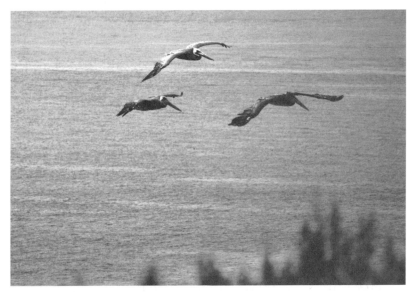

Pelicans soar above—what else?—Pelican Cove.

interpretive center was being built, lead from the bullets had to be flushed out of the soil.

Inside the center are all the usual hallmarks you'd expect: touch tanks, interactive displays, American Indian artifacts, and a gift shop. But the real prize is the wing devoted to Marineland of the Pacific, the former sea-themed amusement park that operated for over thirty years half a mile south of here before closing in 1987. Smaller than San Diego's Sea World but more convenient for Angelenos, the oceanarium boasted a number of famous mammalian residents, including a pilot whale named Bubbles and killer whales Orky and Corky, the latter two re-emerging at Sea World under the name Shamu.

No detail is too trivial for this mini-museum. Amongst its hundreds of collectibles are an original 3-D View-Master with Marineland slides and a matchbook from the park's Porpoise Room Bar and Restaurant, whose spectacularly un-PC emblem was that of a drunken porpoise staggering to stand upright against a lamppost with an empty bottle at his tail—no doubt anchovy-flavored Schnapps.

Next to the Marineland room, find the back door that leads to a patio, which includes a free telescope aimed at the ocean. **Head down the pathway to rejoin the main trail and continue south toward the Point Vicente Lighthouse,** which majestically sprouts out of the landscape in the near distance. Still in use today, the sixty-seven-foot-tall beacon was built in 1926 with a 1,000-watt bulb visible for twenty miles. Its rotating, five-foot lens throws off a reflection that many believe contains the image of a haggard female ghost. Theories differ as to who this "Lady of the Light" is. A former caretaker's lover who fell off the cliffs? A captain's wife awaiting the return of her lost-at-sea husband? An image conjured up after one too many late nights at the Porpoise Room?

The path ends at a dirt parking lot. This is the closest you can get to the lighthouse, which lies on gated-off federal property. It is, however, open for tours on selected Saturdays, so schedule accordingly if you want to see the inside.

Exit the parking lot to pick up the path again by proceeding south along the dirt shoulder of Palos Verdes Drive. After 600 steps on the street, take the turn-off for another parking lot, which overlooks Pelican Cove (marked by a sculpture of a soaring pelican). Find the trail on the west end of the parking lot—it becomes Terranea Trail and continues along the cliff line. The Mediterranean-inspired Terranea Resort will materialize on your left, where Marineland used to be. Though it's one of the more exclusive hotels in Southern California (Frank Vanderlip would be proud), it is surprisingly accessible to non-guests, thanks to public right-of-ways that were established during planning stages.

Stay on the trail until you reach a paved perimeter road, then turn right. After a few steps, you'll hit your halfway point—Nelson's, a cozy restaurant named after Lloyd

Bridges's character in the TV show *Sea Hunt*, which filmed at Marineland. Snag an outdoor table near a fire pit. As you dig into mahi-mahi tacos and take in views

EXTRA STEPS

South of Nelson's, Terranea Trail descends to tide pools below the hotel. The Pelican Cove parking lot has a good map of all the trails in the area, as does Terranea Resort.

of Catalina across the white-capped Pacific, you forget about your walk back and find yourself counting down the minutes to happy hour as you scheme up reasons to stay in Palos Verdes forever.

52

SAN PEDRO

WHERE L.A. GOES SOUTH

This loop favors San Pedro's hilly waterfront, covering two historic lighthouses, one really big bell, and a neighborhood that's fallen off the face of the earth. But fear not—by the time you climb your way into an old machine-gun nest, victory will be yours!

- **TERRAIN:** Flat with gradual and moderate inclines, with one short, steep incline
- **SURFACE:** Mostly paved
- **FIDO FRIENDLY?:** Yes
- **PARKING:** Lot for 22nd Street Park, 22nd Street, San Pedro, across from the Cabrillo Beach Yacht Club

San Pedro is the Rodney Dangerfield of Los Angeles communities. Its Port of Los Angeles is one of the busiest harbors in the nation, substantially contributing to the city's economy. Its military installations have played vital roles in defending our homeland. It boasts the last remaining Warner Grand Theatre still in operation in the Southland, and it gave rise to the best punk band to ever come out of L.A.— the Minutemen. Yet somehow, it gets no respect. Maybe that's because it's so far away from the rest of Los Angeles, hanging by the thread known as Harbor Gateway so that L.A. could have its own deep-water harbor. Whatever the case, today we cast a strong Vote for Pedro.

Begin at the parking lot of the 22nd Street Park. As part of an image makeover, San Pedro is in the process of redeveloping much of its industrial waterfront. This eigh-

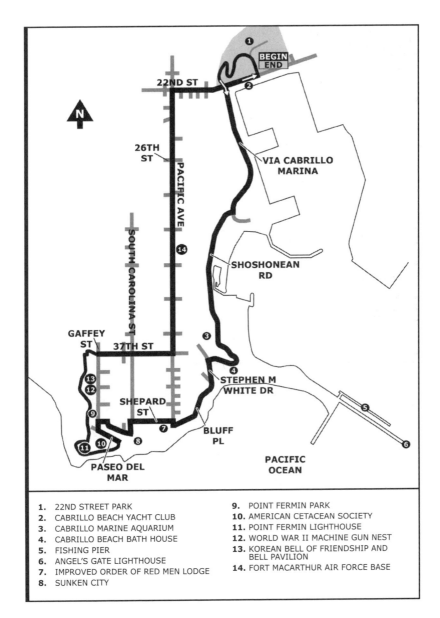

1. 22ND STREET PARK
2. CABRILLO BEACH YACHT CLUB
3. CABRILLO MARINE AQUARIUM
4. CABRILLO BEACH BATH HOUSE
5. FISHING PIER
6. ANGEL'S GATE LIGHTHOUSE
7. IMPROVED ORDER OF RED MEN LODGE
8. SUNKEN CITY
9. POINT FERMIN PARK
10. AMERICAN CETACEAN SOCIETY
11. POINT FERMIN LIGHTHOUSE
12. WORLD WAR II MACHINE GUN NEST
13. KOREAN BELL OF FRIENDSHIP AND BELL PAVILION
14. FORT MACARTHUR AIR FORCE BASE

teen-acre grassy area used to hold storage tanks for the Union Oil Company, while in the northeast corner, a World War II-era warehouse has been converted to an artisan marketplace and brewhouse.

To get a flavor of the park, take the trail to the right of the bocce ball courts. Go left at the fork, following the path as it returns you to the lot. Next, head west on 22nd Street, then cross over to Via Cabrillo Marina. To your left, you'll find rows of masts from Holiday Harbor Cabrillo Marina. **As the street gradually curves westward, turn right at the blue sign advertising Cabrillo Beach and the Aquarium, onto Shoshonean Road.** After 600 steps, you'll reach a ticket booth for a parking lot. Motorists are required to take a ticket. You are a walker. Nod and wink at the hapless drivers as you breeze through the sidewalk to the right of the booth.

On your left, you'll see San Pedro's only white sandy beach; on your right, the Cabrillo Marine Aquarium, an excellent marine nature center. **Shuffle past the lawn to the lot's roundabout,** which hosts a WPA-era statue of explorer Juan Rodriguez Cabrillo, the first European to lay eyes on San Pedro Bay. Nearby is the Cabrillo Beach Bath House. The historic landmark is the last of many bath houses that used to dot SoCal's beaches. Served by the Pacific Red Line, it rented suits and towels for ten cents and was even used for the 1932 Olympic Games. Behind the bath house is a hidden fishing pier that is truly unique. With views of the Los Angeles Harbor, it's the only straight-line pier in Los Angeles to face away from the ocean.

Exiting the parking lot, you'll come to a traffic island with a statue of a bearded dude saluting you. Pay your respects to Mr. Stephen M. White, who, if his epitaph is to be believed, literally died trying to secure San Pedro as Los Angeles's official harbor against rival Santa Monica Bay's losing bid.

Head south on Stephen M. White's namesake street (it's the one to the left of his monument) and continue straight ahead on Bluff Place. Envy the smallish homes with million-dollar ocean views that you will never have. Note the Angel's Gate Lighthouse at the end of the breakwater in the distance, braving nature's elements since 1913.

Continue on Bluff until it makes a sharp right turn, then quickly go left on Shepard Street. At 543 Shepard is a 100-year-old Craftsman

house whose sign displays a red American Indian over the words "Wigwam Sequoia Tribe No. 140." The lodge has nothing to do with American Indians; it belongs to the Improved Order of Red Men. Founded during the American Revolution, it claims to be the country's oldest fraternal organization (and clearly the one with the most outdated name).

Turn left on South Carolina Street. At the end of the block, find the "End" sign as the road veers right into a quasi-alleyway. Beyond the sign is an abandoned neighborhood that gradually fell into the ocean starting in 1929, earning it the nickname Sunken City. Despite a fence, the forbidden grounds have become a haven for partiers and the curious. A word of warning: Sunken City continues to sink and is dangerous to navigate. However, should a sudden squall lift you off your feet and deposit you inside as it did me, a graffiti-laden dystopia awaits you—weeping palm trees, flipped-over foundations, and crumbled concrete streets with exposed pipes and manhole covers hovering over a rocky shoreline.

Continue west along the alley until it rejoins Shepard. On the corner of Shepard and Gaffey Street is a grassy island with military installations marking the entrance to Point Fermin Park. If you're hankering for a meal, join the friendly biker crowd at the appropriately-named Walker's Café, a Pedro institution just a few steps

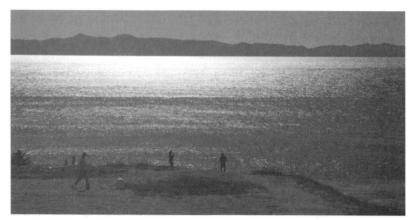

Catalina Island looms in the distance in this majestic view from Point Fermin.

away on Paseo Del Mar.

Access the walking trail at the south end of the park above the bluffs, which offers more views of Sunken City. After passing the American Cetacean Society (a conservation group that pioneered whale-watching boat trips), the path leads to the Point Fermin Lighthouse, a rare Stick style Victorian gem from 1874 (guided tours are offered in the early afternoon). With its decorative railings, gabled roof, and front porch custom-made for sipping lemonade, it looks more like a *house* more than a lighthouse. That was just fine for the husband-and-wife keepers who once lived here with their eight children. The beacon went dark during the imposed blackouts of World War II and is no longer used.

Follow the park's pathway to its north end. Cut over to the sidewalk of Paseo Del Mar and follow that street east back to Gaffey. Turn left, crossing Shepard. Access the parking lot driveway and proceed to the foot trail at the northwest edge of the lot. Huff and puff up the small but steep hill in front of you. Trust me, it's worth the climb.

About 150 steps up, you'll come across an abandoned machine gun nest, like something out of *Saving Private Ryan*. Its cavity is accessible for climbing into. It's one of many shelters, tunnels, munition storages, and missile trackers that still pepper this hillside from its days as a military base for World War II.

Another 150 steps will take you to a sealed-off bunker on the western slope. The fear of a Japanese attack weighed heavily on SoCal's beachside communities, many of which built similar bunkers. And for good reason. A few weeks after the Pearl Harbor bombing, a Japanese submarine torpedoed the SS *Absaroka* just off of Point Fermin, killing a crewman.

Fittingly, the top of the bulge brings a monument to peace in the form of the Korean Bell of Friendship and Bell Pavilion, which has emerged as San Pedro's greatest icon. The seventeen-ton bell was gifted in 1976 by South Korea and honors veterans of the Korean War. Its intricate engravings include several Lady Liberty figures with a Korean counterpart. The bell tolls only four times a year, including Independence Day and Korean Liberation Day. There's always a nice westerly breeze up here, drawing kite-fliers and model plane hobbyists. Gazing out into the Catalina Channel with the bell's pavilion in the foreground will give you perhaps the most spiritual ocean vista in all of Los Angeles.

Exit the parking lot's driveway just north of the bell. A crosswalk will take you to 37th Street. Walk two blocks to Pacific Avenue and turn left, staying on the right sidewalk. It's about 1,800 steps back to 22nd Street. Most of this stretch passes by Fort MacArthur Air Force Base. Keep an eye out for the commemorative marker a few steps past 26th Street, visible through the wrought-iron fence.

When you hit 22nd Street, turn right. Proceed 600 steps to the parking lot for the 22nd Street Park. Ports O'Call—San Pedro's old-school waterfront district—is a mere mile from here. If you haven't worked up an appetite for a bucket of clams and a frosty cold ale after a mountainous five-mile walk, when else will you?

ACKNOWLEDGMENTS

This book is first and foremost a love letter . . . to Los Angeles. But then, you already know that. What you don't know is that I owe a huge debt of gratitude to my mother Marion, who showed me how to walk in both the literal and spiritual sense. She was the first one to open my eyes to the wonders of my native city, and encouraged me and my siblings to seek adventures in the then-unspoiled wilderness behind our Betty Lane house, as long as we were home by dinner time.

I also want to thank my wife Suzie for her endless support throughout the process of researching and writing this book. I am very fortunate to have found a life partner who shares my restless soul yet keeps our family firmly grounded. Suzie and our children are the reasons *why* I walk.

There are so many others who contributed to this book. I would literally be lost without Google Maps, which I relied on almost exclusively to help me chart out my walks. I was also aided by hundreds of books, newspaper articles, and websites, which I leaned on heavily for city history. I found the *Los Angeles Times* archives and KCET's website to be particularly helpful. The Santa Monica Mountains Conservancy, the Los Angeles Conservancy, and Hollywood Heritage are just some of the preservation-minded organizations that also provided a lot of answers. I have long admired the tireless and often thankless work they do as stewards for L.A.'s urban and natural riches.

Then there are those individuals who helped shape this book simply by living inspiring lives. Huell Howser taught me that virtually every mundane landmark in California can be "amaaaazing!" if you simply look at it the right way. A former neighbor, Sol Shankman, showed me that the key to living well into your nineties was to greet each day like a new beginning. I was privileged to often accompany him and soak up his wisdom during his daily hikes into Griffith Park. Speaking of which, the first time I met former councilman Tom LaBonge was near Mount Hollywood, when he told me to "go long" and threw a football into my fumbling hands. LaBonge's enthusiasm for the City of Angels was unrivaled by any other elected official. His well-tread motto to "continue to enjoy and love Los Angeles" are words every Angeleno should live by. Finally, shouts out to Sydnee Davidson, David Carlson, Ray Dean, and Jeff and Darah Kabot (our cover models!) for helping me with aspects of this book.

And, of course, special thanks to the staff at Santa Monica Press, particularly publisher Jeffrey Goldman and his trusty cohort Kate Murray. They provided the essential final steps to giving these walks a life for all to enjoy.

ABOUT THE AUTHOR

Paul Haddad is the author of *Skinny White Freak*, an illustrated young adult novel about bullying, and *High Fives, Pennant Drives, and Fernandomania: A Fan's History of the Los Angeles Dodgers (1977–1981)*, which received praise from the *Los Angeles Times*, ESPN Radio, NBC, CBS, American Public Media, and several other media outlets. A graduate of USC's School of Cinematic Arts, Haddad writes and directs documentaries for the National Geographic Channel and Discovery Networks. Before becoming an avid walker, Haddad was a long-distance bicyclist with a set goal of several "century rides" (100 miles in a day) per year. He has cycled most of the California coast and much of Ireland, and circumnavigated the Big Island of Hawaii, an experience he wrote about for *L.A. Sports & Fitness*.

Haddad lives in Los Feliz with his wife and two children. He starts most days with a hike into Griffith Park with his dog, Porter, who regards horse troughs as random baths placed there for his enjoyment.

Proceeds from each book sale of *10,000 Steps a Day in L.A.* will be donated by the author to TreePeople and the Los Angeles Conservancy.